# FLORENCE NIGHTINGALE
## *She Dared to be Different*

*A lady with a lamp shall stand
In the great history of the land,
A noble type of good,
Heroic womanhood.*
　　*Henry Wordsworth Longfellow
　　　　(1807–1882)*

# FLORENCE NIGHTINGALE
## *She Dared to be Different*

**Second Edition**

**Pushpa Biswas** RNRM BSc (Nursing)
Former Chief Matron
Kasturba Health Society, Kasturba Hospital
Mahatma Gandhi Institute of Medical Sciences
Sevagram, Wardha, Maharashtra, India

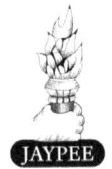

**JAYPEE BROTHERS MEDICAL PUBLISHERS**
*The Health Sciences Publisher*
New Delhi | London

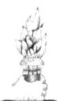 **Jaypee Brothers Medical Publishers (P) Ltd**

### Headquarters
Jaypee Brothers Medical Publishers (P) Ltd
EMCA House, 23/23-B
Ansari Road, Daryaganj
New Delhi 110 002, India
Landline: +91-11-23272143, +91-11-23272703
+91-11-23282021, +91-11-23245672
Email: jaypee@jaypeebrothers.com

### Corporate Office
Jaypee Brothers Medical Publishers (P) Ltd
4838/24, Ansari Road, Daryaganj
New Delhi 110 002, India
Phone: +91-11-43574357
Fax: +91-11-43574314
Email: jaypee@jaypeebrothers.com

### Overseas Office
J.P. Medical Ltd
83 Victoria Street, London
SW1H 0HW (UK)
Phone: +44 20 3170 8910
Email: info@jpmedpub.com

### EU GPSR Authorised Representative
Logos Europe, 9 rue Nicolas Poussin
17000, La Rochelle, France
Phone: +33 (0) 6 67 93 73 78
E-mail: Contact@logoseurope.eu

Website: www.jaypeebrothers.com
Website: www.jaypeedigital.com

© 2024, Jaypee Brothers Medical Publishers

The views and opinions expressed in this book are solely those of the original contributor(s)/author(s) and do not necessarily represent those of editor(s) and publisher of the book.

All rights reserved. No part of this publication may be reproduced, stored or transmitted in any form or by any means, electronic, mechanical, photocopying, recording or otherwise, without the prior permission in writing of the publishers.

All brand names and product names used in this book are trade names, service marks, trademarks or registered trademarks of their respective owners. The publisher is not associated with any product or vendor mentioned in this book.

Medical knowledge and practice change constantly. This book is designed to provide accurate, authoritative information about the subject matter in question. However, readers are advised to check the most current information available on procedures included and check information from the manufacturer of each product to be administered, to verify the recommended dose, formula, method and duration of administration, adverse effects and contraindications. It is the responsibility of the practitioner to take all appropriate safety precautions. Neither the publisher nor the author(s)/editor(s) assume any liability for any injury and/or damage to persons or property arising from or related to use of material in this book.

This book is sold on the understanding that the publisher is not engaged in providing professional medical services. If such advice or services are required, the services of a competent medical professional should be sought.

Every effort has been made where necessary to contact holders of copyright to obtain permission to reproduce copyright material. If any have been inadvertently overlooked, the publisher will be pleased to make the necessary arrangements at the first opportunity.

**Inquiries for bulk sales may be solicited at:** jaypee@jaypeebrothers.com

*Florence Nightingale: She Dared to be Different*

*First Edition:* 2010

*Second Edition:* **2024**

ISBN: 978-93-5696-642-0

Dedicated to the Values, Vision, and Spirit of Florence Nightingale

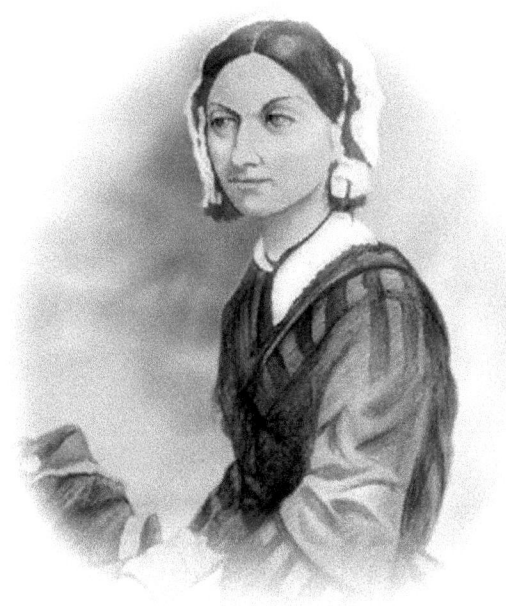

Born May 12th, 1820
Died August 13th, 1910

"All glory comes from daring to begin."

**William Shakespeare**

# Preface to the Second Edition

**Nursing is love in action.**

Why we are functioning at all !
What we want to be efficient for!

**Love is the fundamental energy of the human spirit, the fuel on which we run, the well spring of our vitality**

### The concept of 'Caring Care' in Nursing

The galloping changes in the healthcare delivery is demanding that the care which is meted out to the sick, should be more responsible, more empathetic and more caring.

Sickness magnifies a person's dependency on others. The sick person is more and more in need of attention, understanding and tender care.

Care today is more disease-oriented and healthcare workers concentrate more on the 'disease' and less on the person who is sick. Ivan Illich, the philosopher calls this 'the medicalization of life'.

Florence Nightingale practiced bedside, individualized, transpersonal care. Nurses have inherited from her the concept of 'care' in a cure-dominated-system. Are we (nurses) losing our grip on this rich heritage?

Technology is increasing by leaps and bounds, specializations in nursing have taken precedence over the general bedside nursing—more and more nurses have moved away from the bedside and have allowed machines and gadgets to come in between them and the patient—no one is against technology, neither am I, nor am I against nurses being 'high-tech', but in the race to be high-tech we have forgotten that the prime role and responsibility of a nurse is to be a 'high-touch specialist' we have to remember—always that **'the core of nurses work is care'**.

This book is a small endeavor to bring back nurses to the bedside, to awaken their **'love for caring'**, to enable them to accept the challenges of bedside care and to enjoy the special uniqueness of being a bedside nurse. The time has come to value and embrace the caring practices and expert knowledge and skills that are an important part of nursing practice.

**Pushpa Biswas**

# Preface to the First Edition

*Dear Readers*
What started out as a fascination, soon turned into a passion, as over the years, I collected matter related to Florence Nightingale. There were days when I thought of nothing else.

When I decided to compile all the collected matter, it was not easy. I delved into all old diaries and notebooks; every little scrap of paper, all jottings and scribblings were carefully read and recorded. The old saying which my mother often repeated— 'anyone who can read, can never clean up an attic,' proved to be a boon, for I had not thrown away old diaries and notebooks. I also delved through 'History of Nursing,' especially the events of the 19th century. What I had in the form of a book was 'Notes on Nursing' by Florence Nightingale herself plus some articles on her life. The curiosity to know more about her life made me open encyclopedias, biographies and, of course, search the Internet. I had organized exhibitions on the life of Florence Nightingale for my nurses and so I had some material to start with, but it was not enough.

This compilation is, therefore, a very small section of her life-events and the readers can keep adding whatever comes their way and plenty will, since a strong effort is being made to make everything she wrote, available through electronic publishing.

With best wishes

**Pushpa Biswas**

"Dream what you dare to dream, go where you want to go. Be what you want to be."

# The Ministering Angel

They lay there by the hundreds
and she alone:
Lamp in hand, traversed
the four miles of beds at night.
Yearning to nurse them all;
Her heart reached out to the men
Writhing in agony and pain;
She stooped to caress a fevered brow
To wipe away sweat,
To change a sheet,
To dress a wound,
To hold a hand,
To console a weeping lad.

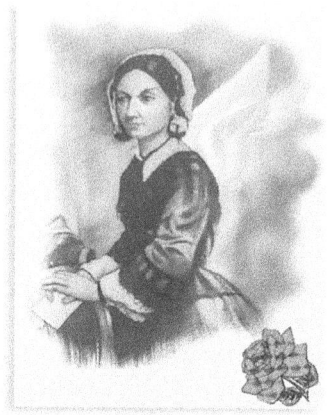

She had, had a long day
The night would be longer;

She stopped by those
Who would not see the morn
A last message, a last wish
Something for the family!

For her nursing was sacred
In her own words a 'Serenifer'

**Pushpa Biswas**

# Acknowledgments

*"Gratitude is the memory of the heart".*

- To my 'Ishta Devta' for all the productive moments so generously given to me.
- To my mother, whose unwavering support guided me into the noble vocation of nursing when I was an uncertain teenager.
- To my beloved husband, Shri Shekhar Thakur, whose ever-growing support, affection, and nurturing care have been my steadfast companions, and for the vast collection of books that enrich my library.
- To my daughter Vinita Singh, for her consistent caring and support. I cherish her.
- To my family, friends and to all those in this caring profession.
- To M/s Jaypee Brothers Medical Publishers (P)Ltd, especially Shri Jitendar P Vij (Group Chairman), Mr Ankit Vij (Managing Director), Mr MS Mani (Group President), Dr Madhu Choudhary (Director–Educational Publishing), Ms Pooja Bhandari [Director–Production (Books and Journals)], Mr Ajay Kumar Sharma [Deputy General Manager (Books and Journals)], Ms Sunita Katla (Executive Assistant to Group Chairman and Publishing Manager), Ms Samina Khan (Executive Assistant to Director–Educational Publishing), Ms Jitika Royal (Content Strategist–Nursing), Mr Rajesh Sharma (Production Coordinator), Ms Seema Dogra (Cover Visualizer), Ms Neha Verma (Graphic Designer–Cover), Mr Rahul Jadli (Proofreader), Mr Akshay Thakur (DTP Typesetter), Mr Radhey Shyam (Graphic Designer) and their team members, who are a 'silent blessing' and without whom this book would not be in your hands.

*A grateful mind is*
*A great mind which*
*Eventually attracts to*
*Itself great things.*

**Plato**

# Contents

1. Introduction — 1
2. Florence Nightingale: The Saint — 4
3. Florence Nightingale: The Statistician — 6
4. Florence Nightingale: The Writer — 8
5. Florence Nightingale: The Linguist — 15
6. Florence Nightingale: The Educationist — 16
7. Florence Nightingale: The Sanitarian, The Hygienist and Hospital Reformer — 19
8. Florence Nightingale: Nurse Administrator and Nurse Manager: A Woman of Action — 22
9. Florence Nightingale: The Epidemiologist — 23
10. Florence Nightingale: The Nutritionist — 24
11. Florence Nightingale: The Feminist — 26
12. Florence Nightingale: The Humanitarian, The Nurse — 32
13. Glorious Tributes to 'A Ministering Angel' — 36
14. Did You Know? — 43
15. Letters — 45
16. We Know Now, What Was Not Known Then — 49
17. Nurses Corner — 51
18. Important Dates and Events — 109
19. Priceless Pearls: Quotations of Miss Florence Nightingale — 116
20. Strange but True — 122
21. Apprehensions — 123
22. India—Florence Nightingale's Vision and Contributions — 125
23. Caring is Active Prayer — 128
24. Conclusion — 136

*Further Reading* — *139*
*Index* — *141*

# CHAPTER 1

# Introduction

> Poetry and imagination begin life. A child will fall on its knees on the gravel walk at the sight of a pink hawthorn in full flower, when it is by itself, to praise God for it."
> —Florence Nightingale—

Today when the nursing profession is an established, scientific, organized profession we cannot help but remember with deep gratitude, contributions made by this great lady—the greatest nurse of all times, the founder of Modern Nursing, Florence Nightingale.

At a time when it was unthinkable for aristocracy to send their women out to pursue professions, certainly not nursing, she dared to be a nurse—she dared to be different.

## A CHILDHOOD IN THE LAP OF LUXURY, YET DIFFERENT

Florence's childhood was spent in the lap of luxury, with numerous servants at her beck and call, two big houses surrounded by acres of gardens to live and play in and indulgent parents who took her and her sister Parthenope to see the splendors of the European countries.

## HER FAMILY

> "Try making your life into a daring adventure."

## THE FATHER DAUGHTER SPECIAL BOND— A BOND WITH A DIFFERENCE

Education brought Florence and her father together. Florence's intellectual self-confidence was a gift given by her father.

# Chapter 1: Introduction

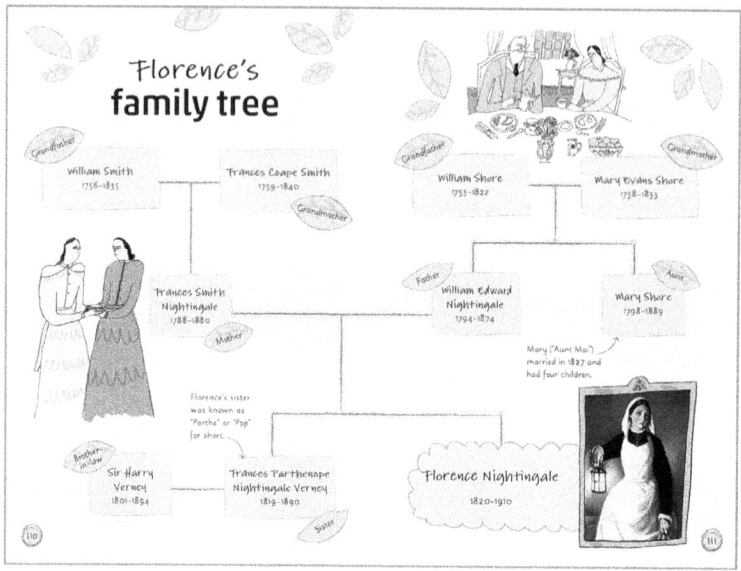

Her father had progressive ideas about women's education. He personally supervised the education of both his daughters, and a governess was always a part of the Nightingale household.

Her sister's interests lay in painting and needlework and writing, Florence was academically oriented.

## A SOUND, COMPREHENSIVE BUT AN EDUCATION WITH A DIFFERENCE

Florence excelled in mathematics and had a special interest in statistics, in which her father was an expert.

Her father tutored her in German, Latin, Greek, Mathematics, Science, Philosophy and politics. She also learnt other languages like French, Italian from her father. Her father's Greek was excellent and he was a great admirer of Plato. Greek is much harder than French or even Latin it was under his influence that at the age of sixteen she had read a good deal of Homer and the Phaedo, the Crito, and the Apology by Plato in the original, she continued to study Greek well into her twenties and soon had a good command of the language.

Chapter 1: Introduction

*"Tutored in Mathematics from her father and aunt and also by James Sylvester."*

She pursued knowledge with great appetite and was extremely focused and confident.

Florence's 'brilliancy' was the 'special bond' that brought her very close to her father.

As Florence puts it, "When I was ten my mother would have no more governesses and my father took us himself in hand. He taught me Latin and Greek and Mathematics and whatever he knew himself. I had the most enormous desire of acquiring—for seven years of my life. I thought of little else but the cultivation of my intellect. And even now when I think what a human intellect may become by industry, ambition comes before me like Circe with her cup to tempt me."

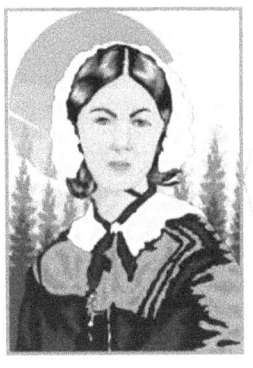

> Florence Nightingale was more confident in her intellectual ability than almost any other woman in England (of her generation)

> This multifaceted approach endeavors to lift a little of the myth and mystery that surrounds this formidable and enigmatic person

> In 1870 Benjamin Jowett asked her comments on the introduction to the translations of the dialogues of Plato (which brought him fame and acclaim)

> Her intellectual training as well as her intellect set her apart from other female contemporaries—she was accepted both as colleague and adversary by men in real world affairs

## THE CALLING

It is said of the first hermits—

"They dwelt in the desert where the air was more pure and the heaven more open and God more familiar."

In a world which is daily growing noiser, and louder, the duty of the civilized man is to have moments of thoughtful stillness as Lord Krishna in the Bhagavad Gita insists that the 'seeker' should be alone to feel the gentle pressure, to hear the quiet voice.

# CHAPTER 2

## Florence Nightingale: The Saint

> "Your sacred space is where you can find yourself again and again."
> —Joseph Campbell—

Florence Nightingale was brought up in a deeply religious family and felt very close to God, even as a small child. She wrote in her private notes that on three different occasions she heard the voice of God calling her to his service.

In 1837, while walking in the garden at Embley, Florence received what she was to later describe as her "calling". She heard the voice of God calling her to do his work. She realized that her mission in life was to serve the sick.

Her sister Parthenope said that Florence had the greatest natural intense love of God and that she did not care at all for individuals, only for the whole race of God's creatures.

Nightingale did not believe that God wanted or intended men to suffer, and she was fiercely convinced that the job of a nurse was to relieve the physical suffering of others, not to save her own soul by tending the sick.

She was a mystic at heart. She read and was influenced by the Catholic mystics, specially St. John of the Cross and St. Theresa.

> "The mystical state is the essence of common sense."
> FN

Her mysticism was not passive:

> "Religion is not devotion but work and suffering for the love of God."
> FN

## Chapter 2: Florence Nightingale: The Saint

"The way to live with God is to live with ideas—not merely to think about ideas but to do and suffer for them."

FN

"There will be no heaven, unless we make it."

FN

"Must we not 'Possess' God here, if we want to 'Possess' him hereafter."

FN

"Desire for personal salvation is not religion."

FN

"Oh God, let me not sink in these perplexities but give me a great cause to do and die for (Private Note)."

FN

# CHAPTER 3

# Florence Nightingale: The Statistician

> "The past informs the future."
> —Pearl Buck—

> Karl Pearson acknowledged Nightingale as a "Prophetess" in the development of applied statistics.

*Florence Nightingale: A pioneer in the visual presentation of information.*

## INTRODUCTION

A little known aspect of Florence Nightingale's life is her achievement in the field of statistics. She invented a diagram she called the 'coxcomb'—better known today as the 'pie chart'.

Florence had an excellent mind and insisted on taking classes with a science background for her learning needs exceeded counting linen, studying French, and enjoying theater arts, Florence was proficient in accounting, and quickly mastered statistical analysis. These were nontraditional educational experiences for a young woman of her standing, but as Florence made it clear to her mother on more than one occasion that 'needlework' was not what she wanted to do.

> Florence was different—she dared to be different.

## PIE

**PIE:** Acronym for a process-oriented documented system. The progress notes in the patient record use.

**Chapter 3:** Florence Nightingale: The Statistician

P — to define the particular problem;
I — to document intervention; and
E — to evaluate the patient outcome.
PIE charting integrates care planning with program notes.

Use of the pie chart—to depict changing patient outcomes. She used this method in the military field hospital that she managed.

She also developed a Model Hospital Statistical Form for hospitals to collect and generate consistent data and statistics.

She was the first female member of the Royal Statistical Society. This membership was attained in 1858 and then in 1874 she became honorary member of the American Statistical Association.

Florence Nightingale revolutionized the idea that social phenomena could be objectively measured and subjected to mathematical analysis. She was an innovator in the collection, tabulation, interpreter, and graphical display of descriptive statistics.

## THE STATE OF STATISTICAL SCIENCE IN FLORENCE NIGHTINGALE'S TIME

There was a great revolution in this area in Nightingale's time. In 1837, the General Registry Office at Somerset House, led by William Farr who later helped Florence with her Crimean Statistics, began to systematically record births, deaths, and marriages in the UK. This gave people the opportunity to examine new cause and effect relationships using registration statistics.

Part of Florence Nightingale's interest in statistics was related to her Unitarian faith. Unitarians believe that mankind has the power to continuously improve itself by observation and the use of reason.

After the Crimean War (1854-56), Florence Nightingale created a number of spectacular graphics designed to show how improvements in building hygiene could save many lives. These appear in five different documents:
1. Appendix 72 of the report of the Royal Commission by Florence Published 1858.
2. Mortality of the British Army's 1858.
3. A contribution to the Sanitary History of the British Army (1859).
4. Notes on matter affecting the health of the British Army 1858.
5. England and Her Soldiers—1859 written by Harriet Martineau Florence encouraged Martineau to write about the war.

CHAPTER 4

# Florence Nightingale: The Writer

> 'The pen is the tongue of the mind'.
> —Cervantes—

> In 1844, she said she would 'so much rather live than write, writing is only a supplement to living.' But the sheer amount that came from her pen is enormous.

Many of her writings represent months of unceasing labor and all reflect deep care and thought in their composition unluckily for nurses very little of what she wrote is available for study—most of the matter was published in official government reports or in pamphlets or journals.

A lot of great Victorians left an enormous pile of papers behind them so also the 'Nightingales'. It is said of Florence Nightingale that apart from Queen Victoria, she was probably the most prolific woman writer, unfortunately much of her written work remained unpublished and scattered all over the world, often in private collections.

From the age of five Florence started writing down what she was thinking and teaching—she was exceptional, she was different her writings continue to be a valuable resource for nurses, health managers and planners. She campaigned tirelessly to improve health standards.

Her total printed writings, published or privately circulated, are 147 as listed in her biography; 15 of which had been written prior to the publication of her 'Notes on Nursing'.

Chapter 4: Florence Nightingale: The Writer

## NOTES ON NURSING

This book written after approximately 14 years observation of the sick. Florence was 39 years old when the book was published in December 1859.

> "A model of arrangement and brevity".

The 'Notes on Nursing' a slim 136 page book, served as the cornerstone of the curriculum at the Nightingale school and other established nursing schools.

The book was also read widely (and even today) by the general reading public. It was and is considered as a classic introduction to nursing; Notes on Nursing talks about comprehensive bedside care of the sick. An interesting feature to note is that it was not written as a manual to teach nurses to nurse but it was written to assist millions of women who had charge of their families to "think how to nurse".

> The first publication of the 'Notes on Nursing' was in England in December, 1859, by the publisher Harrison. Within a month 15,000 copies were sold—the book appeared in French, Italian, and German in various countries.

## A BRIEF SURVEY OF SOME OF THE MORE IMPORTANT OF FLORENCE NIGHTINGALE'S WRITINGS

> Her Style—Very distinctive, combining as it does an arresting lucidity with a caustic humor which indelibly fix in the reader's mind the thoughts she is expressing.

### Before the Crimean War

**1849**—After a journey to Egypt (with her friends Bracebridges) she printed her 'Letters from Egypt' for private circulation.

**1851**—The small anonymous pamphlet appeared titled 'The institution of Kaiserswerth the Rhine' first work on nursing she ever had printed. It has great historical importance it shows her interest in Fliedners establishment (she called Kaiserswerth her spiritual home).

**1857**—'Notes on matter afflicting the health, efficiency and hospital administration of the British army of the late war'. A lengthy book (least known but a most remarkable work) written at the request of Lord Panmure, Secretary of state for war. When the Royal Commission of 1857 was about to start its labors, and represented the outcome of her observations in the Crimea. It was never published, but in **1858**—At her own expense, it was printed for private distribution to well-known individuals.

The book was composed in 6 months Jan-Aug 1857. During this phase, she was not very well. It portrayed her powers of work and profound grasp of the subject. Her careful analysis of all that was lacking assisted the work of 'Royal Commission on the Health of the Army.' These and other books showed Florence Nightingale as an advanced statistician and a pioneer in the use of diagrams or graphs to illustrate the statistics'.

**1859**—Notes on Hospitals—another important book (results of many years of close study of hospitals).

**1860**—Notes on Nursing—American edition the first edition in the US was published by Appleton and Company in 1860.

**1860**—Religious and philosophic matters 'Suggestions for Thought to the Searchers after Truth among the Artizans of England' (printed privately).

**1861**—Abridged form of the 1860 called 'Notes on Nursing' for the laboring classes with a charming additional chapter for girls called 'Minding Baby'.

**1862-1863**—Onwards wrote extensively on India. Her contributions began with a 'Report of the Royal Commission on the Sanitary State of the Army in India'. She continued to write for 30 years on matters affecting Indian health and hygiene. In these, she writes as a SANITARIAN rather than a nurse and shows herself far ahead of her contemporaries regarding preventive medicine.

**1871**—'Introductory Notes on Lying in Institutions', an important book on a subject allied to nursing.

## Chapter 4: Florence Nightingale: The Writer

**1882**—Her most interesting articles contributes (in 1882) to Quains Dictionary of medicine entitled 'Nurses, Training of, and Nursing the Sick'—wherein she formulates her views on nurse training in greater detail than anywhere else and shows us as always her high ideals for nurses.

Voluminous correspondence on many topics with persons all over the world. Benjamin Jowett (1817-1893) Master of Balliol College, Oxford; with whom for a long period she exchanged letters on philosophical and religious subjects.

An annual letter to the nurses of the Nightingale school. Setting forth her own unchanging ideals. These are preserved in the Nightingale school; A few are in the British Museum.

Miss Pringle, at one time Matron of St. Thomas's had some 200 letters from Florence Nightingale.

**January 1829**—Undertook her own autobiography in French "La Vie de Florence Rossignol."

**15 publications—They include many on:**
- Nursing
- Hospitals
- Administrations
- Sanitations
- Health

**Other subjects include:**
- Statistics
- Philosophy
- Irrigation
- Protection of aboriginal races
- Famine
- Punishment and discipline
- Conditions in India
- Thrift
- Birds
- Woman suffrage

By reading and rereading her writings one feels that every sentence she wrote is worth quoting.

Edward Cook was the first of Florence Nightingale's biographers to note the extent and variety of her private notes, that is to say, writings where she *addressed largely herself.*

# Chapter 4: Florence Nightingale: The Writer

To nurses 'Florence Nightingale's most interesting book, will always be 'Notes on Nursing, what it is and what it is not' (1859), so arresting in its clear setting forth of the fundamental principles of nursing which remain as true today as when it was first written.'

*Lucy Ridgely Seymer*

'Because these notes (Notes on Nursing) record the skillful observations of a trained eye and mind on the fundamental needs of human being in sickness and in the prevention of sickness, they are to a great degree timeless in their usefulness to the student of nursing in any country in the world.'

*Virginia M Dunbar*

## FLORENCE NIGHTINGALE'S NOTES ON NURSING (A BROAD OUTLINE)

Florence Nightingale believed that every woman is a nurse because every woman, at one time or another in her life, has charge of the personal health of someone.

The focus of nursing knowledge was how to keep the body free from disease or in such a condition that it could recover from disease.

According to Nightingale, nursing ought to signify the proper use of fresh air, light, warmth, cleanliness, quiet, and the proper selection and administration of diet—all at the least expense of vital power to the patient.

That is, she maintained that the purpose of nursing was to put patients in the best condition for nature to act upon them.

### Boundaries of Nursing Practice

- **Ventilation and warming:** The nurse must be concerned first with keeping the air that patients breathe as pure as the external air, without chilling them.
- **Health of houses:** Attention to pure air, pure water, efficient drainage, cleanliness, and light will secure the health of houses.
- **Petty management:** All the results of good nursing may be negated by one defect: not knowing how to manage, what you do when you are there, and what shall be done when you are not there.
- **Noise:** Unnecessary noise, or noise that creates an expectation in the mind, is that which hurts patients. Anything that wakes

## Chapter 4: Florence Nightingale: The Writer

patients suddenly out of their sleep will invariably put them into a state of greater excitement and do them more serious and lasting mischief than any continuous noise, however loud.

- **Variety:** The nerves of the sick suffer from seeing the same walls, the same ceiling, the same surroundings during a long confinement to one or two rooms. The majority of cheerful cases is to be found among those patients who are not confined to one room, whatever their suffering, and the majority of depressed cases will be seen among those subjected to a long monotony of objects about them.
- **Taking food:** The nurse should be conscious of patients' diets and remember how much food each patient has had and ought to have each day.
- **What food?:** To watch for the opinions the patient's stomach gives, rather than to read "analyses of foods," is the business of all those who have to decide what the patient should eat.
- **Bed and bedding:** The patient should have a clean bed every 12 hours. The bed should be narrow, so that the patient does not feel "out of humanity's reach." The bed should not be so high that the patient cannot easily get in and out of it. The bed should be in the lightest spot in the room, preferably near a window. Pillows should be used to support the back below the breathing apparatus, to allow shoulders room to fall back, and to support the head without throwing it forward.
- **Light:** With the sick, second only to their need of fresh air is their need of light. Light, especially direct sunlight, has a purifying effect upon the air of a room.
- **Cleanliness of rooms and walls:** The greater part of nursing consists in preserving cleanliness. The inside air can be kept clean only by excessive care to rid rooms and their furnishings of the organic matter and dust with which they become saturated. Without cleanliness, you cannot have all the effects of ventilation; without ventilation, you can have no thorough cleanliness.
- **Personal cleanliness:** Nurses should always remember that if they allow patients to remain unwashed or to remain in clothing saturated with perspiration or other excretion, they are interfering injuriously with the natural processes of health just as much as if they were to give their patients a dose of slow poison.
- **Chattering hopes and advices:** There is scarcely a greater worry which invalids have to endure than the incurable hopes of

their friends. All friends, visitors, and attendants of the sick should avoid the practice of attempting to cheer the sick by making light of their danger and by exaggerating their probabilities of recovery.

- **Observation of the sick:** The most important practical lesson nurses can learn is what to observe, how to observe, which symptoms indicate improvement, which indicate the reverse, which are important, which are not, and which are the evidence of neglect and what kind of neglect.

**Notes on Nursing**
"This is the work of genius if ever I saw one; it will, I doubt not, create an order of Nurses before it has finished its work."

**Harriet Martineau's Prophesy**

# CHAPTER 5

# Florence Nightingale: The Linguist

> "Language is called the garment of thought."
> —Carlyle Thomas 1795–1881—
> —Scottish historian and essayist—

Florence had a tremendous talent for languages; she learnt to speak French from childhood from her parents and from her mothers French maids; by her late teens she virtually had command of the language. She completed two biographies of Agatha and Christie (her mothers two maids, based on interviews with the young maids).
January 1829 undertook her own autobiography in French.

"La Vie de Florence Rossignol" wrote several letters when she was not even ten to her parents in French.

She learnt Latin from her father before she was eight. Greek had a symbolic value in the 19th century English culture, functioning in many ways as the seal of professional ability and as the distinguishing mark for high caste.

Greek is much harder than French or Latin, but by the age of sixteen Florence had read a good deal of Greek Literature.

Florence Nightingale's superb Greek, her familiarity with not only Plato but her father's favorite Scottish Philosopher, Dugald Stewart, and her command of multiple facts about the world set her apart from her female contemporaries. Besides Greek, French, Latin, she also learnt German. Florence Nightingale's intellectual self-confidence was a gift given by her father.

# CHAPTER 6

# Florence Nightingale: The Educationist

> "An uneducated man who practices physic is justly called a quack, perhaps an imposter. Why are not uneducated nurses called quacks and imposters?"
> —Florence Nightingale—

Florence Nightingale recognized that for England to embrace the idea of women assuming all nursing duties, they needed to be trained professionals, akin to the emerging field of women educators rather than emulating nuns. Confident in her own capabilities and driven by clear objectives, Florence herself exemplified top-tier practical nursing skills, serving as a model for others to emulate and learn from. Influential figures, such as Lord Palmerston, Lord Shaftesbury, and Sidney Herbert not only acknowledged her expertise but also sought her counsel and entrusted her with their confidence. Additionally, Florence hailed from a wealthy family with extensive connections, further bolstering her influence and resources in her endeavors.

Nightingale's plan was to take charge of a hospital or infirmary and there train women supervisors who would revolutionize patient care in the whole of the public hospital system. She had a large circle of reform minded, sanitarian friends who strongly encouraged her to pursue such a plan. She needed their help since she, like all other women in Victorian society, had no qualifications.

In February 1853—she traveled to France—where she had the opportunity to visit all the city's public medical facilities—she attended operations and toured wards. Florence collected "reports, returns, statistics, pamphlets". By this time, she was already putting together the statistical analysis of medical facilities and preparing the questionnaires that were to later form the basis of her work.

## Chapter 6: Florence Nightingale: The Educationist

She rallied for systematic nurses training but did not rate it higher than character—or imagined it to be all sufficient—she was a deeply religions person and for her nursing was a vocation not a trade, but she was an educationist who believed that others besides deaconesses and nuns could be good nurses—she also was a visionary and saw trained nursing as a secular career.

The other point that made the Nightingale School remarkable was its endowment. This is of special interest as showing that Florence Nightingale, whose aim was always educational, very clearly understood the importance of financial independence for the higher interests of such a school. In the words of one writer: 'The distinctive advance made by the Nightingale School was due to its independence. From the first its liberal endowment has allowed it to hold fast its educational ideals. And there it has been proved that the best nursing service in a hospital can be given by pupil nurses of a school that has for its main purpose their education, and not the pecuniary advantage of the hospital.'

This point, gradually lost sight of since Florence Nightingale's day, has only recently been brought again to the attention of those responsible for the training of nurses.

## FLORENCE NIGHTINGALE—THE CARING EDUCATIONIST

Florence Nightingale arranged to provide the soldiers with books, magazines, candles, and a pleasant reading room where they could smoke and drink coffee.

She set up schools for the men in different regiments as well as for the soldiers children. She arranged play reading and lectures. The small army of middle-class reformer volunteers in England, led by Florence's sister Parthenope, was mobilized to acquire—recreational, educational, and decorative materials of every kind.

They sent 1000 copy books, writing material, diagrams, maps, books and music.

Queen Victoria volunteered a print showing "the Duke of Wellington presenting May flowers to little Prince Arthur, his godson." The print was a big success with soldiers.

> Florence Nightingale was determined to collect the knowledge that would help her follow her "calling." In secret, she studied the reports of medical commissions, the pamphlets of sanitary authorities, the histories of hospitals and homes. She spent the intervals of the London season in workhouses.

## FIVE DIFFERENT METHODS OF NURSING THE SICK

Florence Nightingale in notes on hospitals, 1863—five different, 'methods of nursing the sick' which she had seen actually working in various hospitals. Briefly as expressed by her—
1. Where the nurses belong to a religious order, and are under their own spiritual head; the hospital being administrated by a separate and secular governing body.
2. Where the nurses are of a religious order, the head of which administers both order and hospital.
3. Where the nurses are secular under their own head; the hospital having its own separate and secular government.
4. Where the nurses are secular; and under the same secular authority as that by which the hospital where they nurse is governed.
5. Where the nurses are all men and secular, and under the same secular authority as the hospital.

## THE 'NIGHTINGALE' SYSTEM

Three main features established by Florence Nightingale at St Thomas Hospital, subsequently replicated in numerous other healthcare institutions, include:
1. The matron is supreme, she is responsible for the nursing in the hospital, for the kitchen, laundry and domestic staff, for the nursing school and for the appointment and dismissal of the nursing staff. She is answerable only to the Hospital Board.
2. The student nurses 'live in', for their educational and moral good as well as for discipline, their home being attached to the hospital and under the charge of a 'Home Sister'.
3. Theoretical teaching is given to the nurses, including instruction in the basic sciences.

The ward 'sister' occupies a place of great dignity and importance: She is responsible, under the Matron's direction, for the practical teaching of the nurses.

Besides these four fundamental points Florence Nightingale laid great stress on the above-mentioned special distinction of her school, i.e., the independence, financial and otherwise, that it enjoyed owing to its endowment.

She took personal interest in the Nightingale School—She went through the curriculum, questioned nurses and probationers, examined candidates' notes, she interviewed doctors.

# CHAPTER 7

# Florence Nightingale: The Sanitarian, The Hygienist and Hospital Reformer

She was a sanitarian—she wrote, "A healing man who breathed bad air, drank impure water, and was unable to keep his body clean tended to fall ill. If that man was surrounded by thousands of others living in the same conditions, his illness was easily passed on to them."

Florence Nightingale is most remembered as a pioneer of nursing and a reformer of hospital sanitation methods.

In March 1853, Russia invaded Turkey. Britain and France, concerned about the growing power of Russia, went to Turkey's aid. This conflict became known as the Crimean war. Soon after British soldiers arrived in Turkey, they began going down with cholera and malaria.

She took quick action to improve the deplorable condition of the wounded, dramatically reducing mortality rates among soldiers from 40% to 2%.

Nightingale found the conditions in the army hospital in Scutari appalling. The men were kept in rooms without blankets or decent food. Unwashed, they were still wearing their army uniforms that were "stiff with dirt and gore." In these conditions, it was not surprising that in the army hospitals, war wounds only accounted for one death in six. Diseases such as typhus, cholera and dysentery were the main reasons why the death rate was so high amongst wounded soldiers.

She instituted a rational system for receiving and housing the patients as they arrived.
- Men and their linen washed and kept clean
- Brought huge quantities of shirts and sheets so that the linen personal clothing could be changed
- Set up a laundry where the hospital linen would all be boiled to destroy the lice

- Spent hours along with her most skillful nurses washing wounds and changing dressings.

She instructed her nurses to take a clean piece of rag for each patient, not use the same sponge for all the men (as had been the practice of medical officers and orderlies before).

She bought—
- Mops
- Buckets
- Scrubbing brushes
- Soap.

Induced orderlies to clean the wards.

She got the walls whitewashed and the flooring replaced so that it could be scrubbed to keep the vermin's at bay.

Improved the patients' regular diet by directing that:
1. All cooking vessels to be cleaned regularly
2. All meat to be cooked and distributed quickly
3. As many vegetables to be used
4. Constant vigilance and intelligent participation in all aspects of medical care
5. Motivated orderlies and also doctors to be vigilant and alert.

In the history of public health, the 19th century marks turning point Edwin Chadwick (1800-1890) in England published reports focusing the attention of the Government people on the need for sanitary reforms.

By 20th century, the broad foundations of public health *viz*, safe water, clean environment, were laid in all civilized countries.

Florence Nightingale read and was widely influenced by the reports of Edwin Chadwick in that she also later on strove to improve sanitation and hygienic conditions especially in the British Army stationed in India.

> Modern hygiene and sanitation was developed by Sir Edwin Chadwick (1800–1890) and DEA Parkes

## Chapter 7: Florence Nightingale: The Sanitarian, The Hygienist...

Through her research, Nightingale was familiar with the work of doctors like John Snow and public health specialists like Edwin Chadwick. They had established a casual link between disease and contamination most notably between cholera and contaminated water, though they were far from identifying the agents.

> Sir Edwin Chadwick (1800–90), sanitary reformer, head of the New Poor Law Commission (1834–46). Supported Florence Nightingale lobbying for an Indian sanitary commission.

> Sir William Farr (1803–83), pioneering statistician. Became Assistant Commissioner of census returns in 1851 and 1861; Commissioner in 1871. Worked closely with Florence Nightingale in the development of statistics on the causes of mortality.

# CHAPTER 8

## Florence Nightingale: Nurse Administrator and Nurse Manager: A Woman of Action

> "I think one's feelings waste themselves in words; they ought all to be distilled into actions, which bring results."
> —Florence Nightingale—

Florence and her nurses were not allowed entry into the wards for almost a week so they occupied themselves in making shirts, pillows, slings, straw beds, etc.

Out of the 38 nurses that accompanied her to Scutari only 16 were considered by her satisfactory. She enforced rigid rules for the nurses regarding obedience to medical officers—Nurses worked only in wards in which the doctor allowed them—Florence Nightingale exercised endless tact and patience to win the confidence of the medical officers.

She faced staffing problems because of religious conflicts amongst the nurses and so she distributed the Roman Catholics and Protestants as far as possible.

She set up a laundry where she engaged the soldiers wives.

She set up a 'Remittance Scheme' for the soldiers.

## REMITTANCE SCHEME

By which she demonstrated that many soldiers cared about their families and wanted to look after them, although it was not received well Lord Panmure was more annoyed than impressed by the news that Miss Nightingale was sending home money for the men. He felt she was once more poking her nose into army affairs where she had no business.

> 'They who think they can and dare, get new things done.'

CHAPTER 9

# Florence Nightingale: The Epidemiologist

Having worked on a cholera ward, Nightingale knew just how ineffective medical treatment was, and had reached the conclusion that prevention was the best way to approach disease.

Florence Nightingale had done a great deal of serious reading in what might now be called epidemiology, and she had an unusually informed understanding of what was happening at Scutari, e.g., she immediately condemned the standard use in the hospitals of single sponge to wash one man after another, and instructed her nurses to use separate clean rags.

The central issue facing the Army Medical Board in the hospitals at Scutari and Crimea was an epidemic of several infectious diseases, which no one in 1854 understood—it was a matter which the British army officers were unable to understand or handle. Officers of the British army were not sanitarians. In time of war more soldiers died of disease than wounds; however officers considered such losses to be natural and unavoidable. It was left to Florence Nightingale to take up the matter seriously and to bring down the mortality rate within 3 weeks from 42 to 2% but till then hundreds of lives had been lost.

By the end of November 1855 out of a nominal army of 37,232 men, there were 9,003 sick, cholera, dysentery, "Varna fever" and "Crimean fever" mainly were diseases which brought so much disaster and still army officers were not interested in organizing sanitary brigades.

This was the situation that Florence Nightingale found at the Barrack and General Hospital and within weeks of her arrival she had made a difference.

# CHAPTER 10

# Florence Nightingale: The Nutritionist

> Vit C is now known to be essential for the formation of scar tissue and the healing of wounds; Nightingale provided her soldiers plenty of lemons, vinegar and lime juice.

Within 10 days of her arrival in Scutari she had succeeded in establishing a special kitchen where extra diets could be prepared.

Regular digestible and nutritious food was served to the soldiers. She inspected the central kitchen, installed new cooks and instructed the orderlies to be alert and prompt.

Hot soup was served from her own kitchen to the soldiers as and when required.

From her own kitchen she provided soups, beef tea, jellies made from fruits and meat, thin cereal and various concoctions based on wine.

In her book 'Notes on Nursing' she has devoted two whole chapters to what the patient should eat and the problems faced and solutions. In chapter VI 'Taking Food' she says "For instance, to the large majority of very weak patients it is quite impossible to take any solid food before 11 AM, nor then, if their strength is still further exhausted by fasting till that hour."

The food offered should be in accordance with the patients ability to eat or drink, e.g., fever patients—need liquid digestible diet—in chapter VII titled "What Food ?" she talks about in the common errors in diet and the types of diet to be given.

She says—

> "Observation not chemistry, must decide sick diet."

## Chapter 10: Florence Nightingale: The Nutritionist

'Every careful observer of the sick will agree in this that thousands of patients are annually starved in the midst of plenty, from want of attention to the ways which alone make it possible for them to take food.'

**Florence Nightingale 1859**

'Let the patient's taste decide. You will say that, in cases of great thirst, the patient's craving decides that it will drink a great deal of tea, and that you cannot help it. But in these cases be sure that the patients required diluents for quite other purposes than quenching the thirst, he wasn't a great deal of some drink, not only of tea, and the doctor will order what he is to have, barley water or lemonade, or soda water and milk, as the case may be.

**Florence Nightingale 1859**

Many of the foods mentioned by her may not suit and appeal to the Indian setting—but the principles are worth following—

All nurses should read this book with care and should feel responsible for the patient's nutrition.

CHAPTER 11

# Florence Nightingale: The Feminist

> "This system dooms some minds to incurable infancy, others to silent misery" Florence Nightingale (Speaking of the systematic ways in which women's lives and interests were curtailed).

Florence Nightingale faced gender-related difficulties and frustrations. These difficulties and frustrations still exist for women in the developing world and in traditional communities everywhere.

The right of women to fulfill their talents, enter the public sphere, lead independent lives, and freely follow their highest aspirations is still being contested.

After the 'Times Report' Florence Nightingale was asked by the Queen to sail for Crimea:-

## AT SCUTARI

'Not one of those in authority could have been pleased at her coming, since it obviously implied want of confidence in them, and she had to overcome prejudice and opposition from the medical and other officers, themselves often the helpless victims of red tapism.'

## BUT AS NUTTING PUTS IT

'Without the great crisis of the Crimea, the matchless powers of Florence Nightingale might never have been set free, her commanding genius might have found no fitting field for action.'

MA Nutting (a well-known historian)

Coming to nursing there is a definite link between 'Feminism and Nursing'. Not only are most nurses women, but the social role, to care for the sick—of nursing, is one that has been assigned to women all over the world.

Florence Nightingale yearned to pursue a social calling to serve people, but as a Victorian woman she faced severe restriction from her family and society. Here are some quotes which are an outcry against the plight of Victorian women she strongly believed that women had many lost talents and abilities which were curbed because of the restrictions faced in the Victorian era.

## CASSANDRA TROJAN PROPHETESS

Florence Nightingale wrote an essay titled 'Cassandra' but on the advice of her well-wishers it was never published. She picked up the title Cassandra from Greek Mythology—It is believed that Cassandra was given the gift of prophesy by Apollo (Sun God) but was cursed by another God that her prophecies would never be believed by anyone though they would ultimately come true (but too late by then to heed the warnings). Cassandra was the daughter of Priam king of Troy and sister of the mighty Hector (who was killed by Achilles the Greek and whose body he desecrated) and Paris.

Cassandra fore told the doom of Troy when Helen (of Sparta) was abducted by her brother Paris.

The victorious Greek General Agamemnon took Cassandra as his trophy; she prophesied the tragedy that would be fall him (Agamemnon) on his return to Greece.

Today the word 'Cassandra' stands for "a prophet of doom and disaster".

## A FEW EXTRACTS FROM HER ESSAY TITLED 'CASSANDRA'

"What wonder if, wearied out, sick at heart with hope deferred, the springs of will broken, not seeing clearly where her duty lies, she abandons intellect as a vocation and takes it only, as we use the moon, by glimpses through her tight-closed window shutters?

Passion, intellect, moral activity—these three have never been satisfied in woman. In this cold and oppressive conventional atmosphere, they cannot be satisfied. To say more on this subject would be to enter into the whole history of society, of the present state of civilization.

## Chapter 11: Florence Nightingale: The Feminist

When shall we see a life full of steady enthusiasm, walking straight to its aim, flying home, as that bird is now, against the wind with......... calmness and ......... confidence?

If, together man and woman approach any of the high questions of social, political, or religious life, they are said (and justly—under our present disqualifications) to be going "too far" That such things can be !

Yet time is the most valuable of all things, if they had come every morning and afternoon and robbed us of half—a crown, we should have had redress from the police. But it is laid down, that our time is of no value.

Women dream of a great sphere of steady, not sketchy benevolence, of moral activity, for which they would fain be trained and fitted, instead of working in the dark, neither knowing nor registering whither their steps lead, whether farther from or nearer to the aim.

Women ...... long for experience, not patch-work experience, but experience followed up and system to enable them to know what they are about and where they are "casting their bread" and whether it is "bread" or a stone.

With what labor women have toiled to breakdown all individual and independent life, in order to fit themselves for this social and domestic existence, thinking it right ! And when they have killed themselves to do it, they have awakened (too late) to think it wrong.

Nothing can well be imagined more painful than the present position of woman, unless, on the one hand, she renounces all outward activity and keeps herself within the magic sphere, the bubble of the dreams, or, on the other, surrendering all aspiration, she gives herself to her real life, soul and body. For those to whom it is possible, the latter is best, for out of activity may come thought, out of mere aspiration can come nothing.

> And so is the world put back by the death of every one who has to sacrifice the development of his or her peculiar gifts (which were meant, not for selfish gratification, but for the improvement of that world) to conventionality. (1852)

Educated in the liberal tradition by her father. Florence Nightingale wrote "Cassandra in 1852, after she returned from Kaiserworth in Germany (her spiritual home) Cassandra was not published—on

**Chapter 11:** Florence Nightingale: The Feminist

the advice of her well-wishers but later in 1860 it was privately printed—Despite being unpublished her friend John Stuart Mill in his essay on the 'Subjection of Women' 1869 used some ideas from Cassandra Frustrated by the restrictive life of a gentle woman Florence Nightingale ferociously lashes out at the Victorians; here are a few questions, some still need answering".

**Is discontent a privilege?**
Yes, it is a privilege for you to suffer for your race—a privilege not reserved to the Redeemer, and the martyrs alone, but one enjoyed by numbers in every age.

**Why have women passion, intellect, moral activity—these three and a place in society where not one of the three can be exercised?**
Men say that God punishes for complaining. No, but men are angry with misery. They are irritated when women are not happy. They take it as a personal offence. To God alone may women complain without insulting Him!

**When shall we see a woman making a study of what she does?**
Married women cannot, for a man would think, if his wife undertook any great work with the intention of carrying it out—of making anything but a sham of it—that she would "suckle his fools and chronicle his small beer" less well for it—that he would not have so good a dinner—that she would destroy, as it is called, his domestic life.

("Suckling their fools" is a paraphrase of a quotation from Othello—a play by William Shakespeare)

**Is man's time more valuable than woman's?**
Or is the difference between man and woman this that woman has confessedly nothing to do?

> Women are never supposed to have any occupation of sufficient importance not to be interrupted, except "suckling their fools"; and women themselves have accepted this, have written books to support it, and have trained themselves so as to consider whatever they do as not of such value to the world as others, but that they can throw it up at the first claim of social life. They have accustomed themselves to consider intellectual occupation as a merely selfish amusement, which it is their "duty" to give up for every trifler more selfish than themselves.

> The family? It is too narrow a field for the development of an immortal spirit, be that spirit male or female. The family uses people, not for what they are, not for what they are intended to be, but for what it wants for— its own use. It thinks of them not as what God has made them, but as the something which it has arranged that they shall be. This system dooms some minds to incurable infancy, others to silent misery.

## THE FAMILY?

It is too narrow a field for the development of an immortal spirit, be that spirit male or female the chances are a thousand to one that, in that small sphere, the task for which that immortal spirit is destined by the qualities and the gifts which its creator has placed within it, will not be found.

> In one of her letters to her father Florence tells him that she is desperate to escape the bitterness and pain of women—
>
> "Why cannot a woman follow abstractions like a man? Has she less imagination, less intellect, less self-devotion, less religion than a man? I think not."

## I DARE TO BE 'ME'

I dare to be 'me'
I dare to be different
I believe in my convictions
I believe in my dreams;
Being 'true' to myself
Is a maxim I follow,

It helps not to be false to others..........
What others believe I respect.
I dare to be 'me'
I dare to be different.

I know my gifts
I follow my goals
I accept each stress as normal.....
Adversities and failures are feedbacks,
Feedbacks I examine and correct.

## Chapter 11: Florence Nightingale: The Feminist

I'm opportunistic
I make things happen,
I don't lie back and let things happen...
I dare to be 'me'
I dare to be different

I don't sit and yearn for second chances.............
I sit up and take chances....
I am the one—who is in charge of 'me'
I have the power to change
I dare to be 'me'
I dare to be different
I dare to be 'me'
I was meant to be 'me'
I dare to be different
I dare to be 'me'

**P Biswas**

# CHAPTER 12

# Florence Nightingale: The Humanitarian, The Nurse

> The role of nursing as having 'charge of somebody's health' based on the knowledge of "how to put the body in such state to be free of disease or to recover from disease."
>
> —Nightingale 1860—

In the future, which I shall not see, for I am old, may a better way be opened! May the methods by which every infant, every human being will have the best chance of health, the methods by which every sick person will have the best chance of recovery, be learned and practiced! Hospitals are only an intermediate state of civilization never intended, at all events, to take in the whole sick population.

Florence Nightingale—1860

## FORM 'ME' TO 'YOU'

If nurses are to serve the sick, serve the people at large, and serve well—then it has to be an individualistic, humane, holistic approach—the minute we refer to patients as 'clients', as 'customers' as 'consumers', the devotion, dedication, the rapport, the empathy—all fade away and we allow 'health care' to become market-places where people can come and buy health care as a commodity.

Nursing can be called 'nursing' only if it can make a positive difference in the lives of patients and their families, and—make a difference in societies, communities, nations, and the world.

P Biswas

"The World, more especially the hospital world, is in such a hurry, is moving so fast, that it is too easy to slide into bad habits before we are aware".

Florence Nightingale—1873

## Chapter 12: Florence Nightingale: The Humanitarian, The Nurse

### Why have we no Sisters of Charity?
### The Report that changed history.
### The Times October 9 and 12, 1854.

Special correspondent WH Russel described the deplorable condition of the troops, and reported that there were in the hospitals neither surgeons, dressers, nurses, nor the commonest appliances of a workhouse sick ward.

On October 13 he enlarged on this same theme and added that the French troops had the help of 'Sisters of Charity'—His letter the next day boldly demanded 'Why have we no Sisters of Charity?'

This challenge escaped neither Florence Nightingale nor her old friend Sidney Herbert, the Secretary at war.

**Note:** At the outbreak of the Crimean war the Duke of Newcastle was the Secretary for war and Sidney Herbert the Secretary at War.

**The Times October 14, 1854**
The Russians were nursed by Sisters of the Holy Cross Organized by Grand Duchess Elena Pavlovna. There were at one time 200 sisters working for the soldiers.

In the armies of France, the Sisters of Charity had rendered similar services and even ministered to the wounded on the battle field; but their labors were a work of religious charity and not an organized sanitary movement.

**The wounded sick soldiers treated in hospitals:**
- General and the Barrack hospitals (the largest)
- Palace hospital (opened Jan, 1855)
- Hospital at Koulali 4 miles away, opened December, 1854.

**Florence and her nurses were established in the Barrack Hospital.**

The roles that nurses assume today, she adopted and carried out with tremendous dedication and devotion in Crimea. She dealt with soldiers who were under great stress and pain, she dealt with anger and depression, with despair and sorrow with death! As we have seen in the preceding chapters, she was all in one, Administrator, Manager, Leader, Nutritionist, Hygienist, Sanitarian; she served as patient's advocate. Whatever the situation, with whatever available means, (which were very few) in spite of all limitations, she meted out nursing care, demonstrated immense caring and a holistic, humane approach. She was a self-trained nurse yet she was able to deal with as big a crisis as the Crimean war; for her nursing was 'sacred' she was a spiritual person with very progressive ideas—all the knowledge that she had collected over the years—ever since her 'calling' in 1837—she applied with great skill and efficiency—as she carried out the care of the wounded in Scutari she was an educationist and she did not neglect educational needs of the soldiers—I am not going into great details, because in the preceding chapters I have included all the available material regarding her work not only during the war but also during the pre and postwar period.

Florence Nightingale had no fear for her own life and spent many hours a day in Scutari doing individual nursing and she chose to work in fever and dysentery wards. Her skill and sincerity showed in her caring and nursing.

The resources were very scanty and she and her nurses worked from morning till night, and through the night—Today we talk about critical thinking skills—she practiced these skills in crimea; in spite of the nurse shortages (remember they were not trained nurses) she displayed leadership qualities and faced hostile behavior from surgeons and other Army personnel—She worked with the minimum basic requirements (to mete out proper nursing care) and yet managed to bring down the mortality rate from 42/- to a mere 2% that too in a short span. Her sincerity, devotion and skills were demonstrated in her work, in her care and in her humane service.

In short, she was an outstanding nurse, one of the greatest souls that ever lived.

> Her views on nursing were derived from a 'spiritual philosophy'. She viewed nursing as a search for truth in finding answers to health care questions or discovering and using God's law of healing in nursing practice.

> "Without the great crisis of the Crimean, the matchless powers of Florence Nightingale might never have been set free, her commanding genius might have found no fitting field for action......"

## Chapter 12: Florence Nightingale: The Humanitarian, The Nurse

# END OF THE WAR

"I stand at the altar of the murdered men, and while I live I fight their cause."

Peace was finally signed in February 1856, but as the work of the hospitals did not at once cease it was only in August, 1856, that she returned home from Scutari and in the eyes of the world her task was over—In her opinion 'Crimean mission was not so much a climax as an episode' her task had scarcely begun—she was not deterred by her illness the one that started at Balaclava—and although she was advised rest—she continued to work—in her own words—"I stand at the altar of the murdered men, and while I live I fight their cause."

# CHAPTER 13

# Glorious Tributes to 'A Ministering Angel'

Henri Dunant, speech on Florence Nightingale at the Geneva Convection (August, 1864).

To the many who pay their homage to Miss Nightingale, though a very humble person of a small country, Switzerland, I yet want to add my tribute of praise and admiration. As the founder of the Red Cross and originator of the diplomatic Convention of Geneva, I feel emboldened to pay my homage.

To Miss Nightingale I give all the honor of this humane Convention. It was her work in the Crimea that inspired me to go Italy during the war of 1859, to share the horrors of war, to relieve the helplessness of the unfortunate victim to their duty, far from their native country, and to water the poetic land of Italy with their blood.

In 1872, after the Franco-Prussian War, Dunant visited London and read a paper on the work of the society. His first words were these:

"Though I am known as the founder of the Red Cross and the originator of the Convention of Geneva, it is to an Englishwoman that all the honour of that Convention is due. What inspired me to go to Italy during the war of 1859 was the work of Miss Florence Nightingale in the Crimea."

A history of the Western Sanitary Commission, written in 1864, begins with this credit to Florence Nightingale's pioneering work:

The first organized attempt to mitigate the horrors of war, to prevent disease and save the lives of those engaged in military service by sanitary measures and a more careful nursing of the sick and wounded, was made by a commission appointed by the British Government during the Crimean war, to inquire into the terrible mortality from disease that attended the British army at Sebastopol, and to apply the needed remedies. It was as a part of this great work that the heroic young Englishwoman, Florence Nightingale, with her army of nurses, went to the Crimea to care for the sick and wounded soldier, to minister in hospitals, and to alleviate suffering and pain, with a self-sacrifice and devotion that has made her name a household word, wherever the English language is spoken.

Letter in the times on the activities of Florence Nightingale at Scutari (February, 1855).

Wherever there is disease in its most dangerous form, and the hand of the spoiler distressingly nigh, there is that incomparable woman sure to be seen; her benignant presence is an influence for good comfort even amid the struggles of expiring nature. She is a 'ministering angel' without any exaggeration in these hospitals, and as her slender form glides quietly along each corridor, every fellow's face softens with gratitude at the sight of her.

Her method of work was one of untiring thoroughness in reading, assembling, observing, testing and analyzing of everything to be had on the subject at home or abroad, and then lining up her facts with the obvious intent to produce action. Queen Victoria expressed recognition of her thoroughness "I wish we had her at the war office."

## THE NIGHTINGALE PLEDGE

"The Nightingale Pledge" written by Mrs Lystra E. Getter, Superintendent Harper Hospital Detroit, USA in honor of Florence Nightingale in 1893.

I solemnly pledge myself before God
And in the presence of this assembly,
To pass my life in purity and to practice
   My profession faithfully.
I will abstain from whatever is
Deleterious and mischievous and
Will not take or knowingly administer
Any harmful drug.
I will do all in my power to maintain
And elevate the standard of my profession and
Will hold in confidence
All personal matters committed
To my keeping and
All family affairs coming to my knowledge
In the practice of my calling
With loyalty will I endeavour

To aid the physician in his work
And devote myself to the welfare
Of those committed to my care.

**Please Note:** Later, to emphasize the ever-widening field of nursing, Mrs Gretter altered the last clause to:

'With loyalty will I aid the physician in his work, and as a "missioner of health" I will dedicate myself to devoted service to human welfare.'

### 'The Lady with the Lamp'
"Florence Nightingale began to walk the wards at night within days of her arrival at Scutari what began an exploratory tour of inspection turned into a routine and then into a ritual. It symbolized the covenant between her and the men, and they understood its meaning very well."

### LAMP
As we turned the angle of the long corridor to the right, we perceived, at a great distance, a faint light flying from bed to bed, like a will O'the-wisp flickering in a meadow on a summer's eve, which at last rested upon one spot.

**Alexis Soyer**

## To The Lady with The Lamp
### August 13, 1910.

One star still burns albeit the sun declines,
A light goes out, but still one lamp is clear;
The lamp of duty born to persevere
That one time down dark Scutari's noisome lines
Of indescribable agony shone, still shines;
Still dying soldiers feel an angel's cheer,
Content to kiss love's shadow passing near.
And the worst battle woe had anodynes.
Dear lady the lamp so brave, so frail,
The light you lit shall grow to perfect morn
Till wounds no more may need a woman's hand,
Ten thousand thousands in that painless land
To our farewells to-day are crying Hail!
And all the world gives thanks that you were born.

**HD Rawnsley**

## Chapter 13: Glorious Tributes to 'A Ministering Angel'

We think today of the little Russian prisoner, the poor boy who could not speak or be spoken to till she had taken him in and had him taught and made useful; and how he answered when at length he could understand a question. When asked if he knew where he would to when he was dead, he confidently said; "I shall go to Miss Nightingale".

**Harriet Martineau**

**The Bird**
Nightingale 'Singer of the night'
Greek—'filomela'
Persian—'Bulbul'
American—'Thrush'
The soldiers in Crimea affectionately called her "The Bird."

- **The British Soldier's Feeling of Thanks and Reverence of Florence Nightingale**

On a dark lovely night on Crimea's dread shores. There 'd been bloodshed and strife on the morning before:
The dead and the dying lay bleeding around, some crying for help—there was none to be found.
Now God is his mercy. He pitied their cries,
And the soldiers cheerful the morning to rise.

Refrain
So, forward my lads, may your hearts never fail.
You are cheered by the presence of a sweet Nightingale.
Her heart it means good for no bounty she'll take,
She'd lay down her life for the poor soldier's sake;
She prays for the dying, she given peace to the brave,
She feels that a soldier has a soul to be saved.
The wounded they love her as it has been seen,
She's the soldiers preserver, they call her their Queen,

Refrain.
May heaven give her strength and her heart never fail.
One of Heaven's best gift is Miss Nightingale.

What a comfort to see her pass. She would speak to one, nod and smile to as many more; but she could not do it to all you know. We lay there by the hundreds, but we could kiss her shadow as it fell and lay our heads on the pillow again content.

**Anonymous**

## TRIBUTE TO FLORENCE NIGHTINGALE

Gandhiji wrote the following article on Florence Nightingale, which was published in Indian Opinion on September 9, 1915.

"Fifty years ago, the various facilities for nursing the wounded which are available today did not exist, people did not come out to render aid in large number as they do now. Surgery was not as efficacious then as it is today. There were in those days very few men who considered it an act of mercy and merit to succour the wounded. It was at such a time that this lady, Florence Nightingale came upon the scene and did good work worthy of an angel descended from heaven. She was heart-stricken to learn of the sufferings of the soldiers.

Born of a noble and rich family, she gave up her life of ease and comfort to nurse the wounded and the ailing, followed by many other ladies. She left her home on October 21, 1854. She rendered strenuous service in the battle of Inkerman. At that time, there were neither beds nor other amenities for the wounded. There were 10,000 wounded under the charge of this single woman. The death rate among the wounded which was 42%, before she arrived, immediately came down to 31%, and ultimately to 5%. This was miraculous, but can be easily visualized. If bleeding could be stopped, the wounds bandaged and the requisite diet given, the lives of many thousands would doubtless be saved. The only thing necessary was kindness and nursing, which Miss Nightingale provided.

"It is said that she did an amount of work which big and strong men were unable to do. She used to work nearly twenty hours, day and night. When the women working under her went to sleep, she, lamp in hand, went out alone at midnight to the patient's bedside, comforted them, and herself gave them whatever food and other things were necessary. She was not afraid of going even to the battle-front, and did not know what fear was. She feared only God. Knowing that one has to die some day or other, she readily bore whatever hardships were necessary in order to alleviate the sufferings of others."

"This lady remained single all her life, which she spent in good work. It is said that, when she died, thousands of soldiers wept bitterly like little children, as though they had lost their own mother.

No wonder that a country where such women are born is prosperous. That England rules over a wide empire is due, not to the country's military strength, but to the meritorious deeds of such men and women."

**Mahatma Gandhi**

To express her personal appreciation for all Miss Nightingale had done for the troops, Queen Victoria sent her a brooch that Prince Albert himself had designed.

The brooch featured St. George's cross—on which was written "Blessed are the Merciful" and "Crimea".

On the back of the Medal was written: "To Miss Florence Nightingale, as a mark of esteem and gratitude for her devotion towards the Queen's brave soldier's—from Victoria R. 1855".

**If Florence Nightingale be the founder of modern nursing—Sidney Herbert must rank as its patron Sidney Herbert's tribute to Florence Nightingale.**

He paid his tribute by placing of his statue next to that of Florence Nightingale in waterloo place.

It was a brave and original step considering that this step was taken in English mid-nineteenth century!!

## EPOCH-MAKING IDEA

- To have women nurses with the British Army! It was immodest, unthinkable, revolutionary! Yet it was not only suggested but carried into effect.
- The step was bold—but if it had not been taken how different night the history of nursing (have) been !!

[At the outbreak of the Crimean War the Duke of Newcastle was the Secretary for war and Sidney Herbert the Secretary at war.]

Tribute and Acknowledgment of Florence Nightingale's Work.

Queen Victoria, who regarded the army as a primary concern of her own and who ordered that Nightingale's letters be sent to her, once remarked: "We are very much struck by her— wonderful, clear, and comprehensive head. I wish we had her at the war office!"

The sect of the Good Samaritan 'she belongs to a sect which unfortunately is a very rare one the sect of the Good Samaritan'.

**(Clergyman)**

"No, adequate appreciation of Florence Nightingale life can probably yet be written, for like the greatness of hers grows the more striking the further one gets away from it. By nurses she will ever be revered as their Foundress, but this is not all. While she revolutionized nursing she was almost equally great in other fields; her advanced ideas on sanitation or on statistics would alone have entitled her to respect. She remains as one of the most remarkable figures of the 19th Century, Indeed one of the outstanding women of all time."

**Lucy Ridgely Seymer**
[A General History of Nursing]

May 1910 was the Jubilee of the founding of the Nightingale Training School—a meeting was held in New York in the Carnegie Hall at which the Public Orator, Mr Choate, delivered an eulogium on the great record and noble life of Miss Florence Nightingale.

In June 1907—There was a conference held by the 'International Conference of Red Cross Societies' who sent a message to "Miss Florence Nightingale, the pioneer of the first Red Cross Movement, whose heroic efforts on behalf of suffering humanity will be recognized and admired by all ages as long as the world shall last."

Tell Miss Nightingale, that I have endeavoured to follow implicitly everything she has recommended and that I love and respect her more than anyone in the world.

**Grand Duchess of Baden, 1870**

Mark what, by breaking through customs and prejudice, Miss Nightingale has effected for her sex. She has opened to them a new profession, a new sphere of usefulness...... A claim for more extended freedom of action. I do not suppose that in undertaking her mission, she thought much of the effect which it might have on the social position of women. Yet probably not one of those who made that question a special study has done half as much as she towards its settlement.

**Lord Stanley**

# CHAPTER 14

# Did You Know?

- Florence Nightingale had a pet owl called 'Athena'—the owl died when Florence was undertaking preparations to go out to save dying soldiers in the hospital at Scutari.
- Florence Nightingale learnt Greek, Latin and mathematics at the age of ten from her father.
- 4th November 2004 marked the 150th anniversary of Florence Nightingale's arrival at Scutari (Uskudar Turkey).
- When Florence Nightingale had whooping cough her 13 dolls had it too—they were found with pieces of flannel round their necks.
- She wrote her autobiography in French 'La Vie de Florence Rossignol.'
- She invented and established the science of nursing.
- She improved sanitation and hygienic conditions in the British army stationed in India.
- Kaiserswerth Institute in Germany was considered by her as her spiritual home.
- She dreamt of forming a Protestant sisterhood of educated women who could become skillful nurses.
- Florence's pet name was Flo.
- She developed the polar area diagram.
- She was the only woman to receive 'The Order of Merit' by the British Crown.
- She invented a diagram called 'Coxcomb'- better known to—day as the 'Pie Chart.'
- Florence had a beautiful singing voice and had a passion for opera.
- The Nightingale pledge was not written by Florence Nightingale but it was written in honor of Florence Nightingale by Ms Elizabeth Gretter.
- That she was the first practicing nurse epidemiologist.
- She developed a model hospital statistical form to collect and generate consistent data and statistics.

## Chapter 14: Did You Know?

- She never visited India, but so great was her knowledge of Indian sanitary army affairs that no important government official left for India without seeing here.
- She directed the purification of the Madras water system from her bedroom in South Street London.
- She did more work at home than most Cabinet Ministers.
- She never held public office nor any public position after her return from Crimea, but her back bedroom in South Street was referred to as the 'Little war office'.
- Nightingale was the first nursing theorist (she believed the purpose of nursing is to put the person in best condition for nature to restore or preserve health).
- In 1873, Florence Nightingale developed a model for independent nursing schools to teach *Critical Thinking, Attention to Patient's Individual Needs, and Respect for Patient's Rights.*
- She was God Mother to Herr. Fliedner's (Kaiserswerth) child and she educated the child after Fliedner's death in 1864.
- The designate of a 'Home Sister' was first given by Florence Nightingale (This post was created by her for her nursing school).
- She was advisor and organizer for both (when war was declared between) Germany and France in 1870.
- After the Franco-German war, she received both the 'Bronze Cross of the French' and 'Prussian Cross of Merit' from the German Emperor.
- There is a museum in the honor of Florence Nightingale in the Barracks where she worked in what is now part of Istanbul, Turkey.
- She dedicated a lecture on 'Sick Nursing and Health Nursing', to Princess Christian.
- She erected a 20 feet high marble cross—to the fallen soldiers on a mountain peak above Balaclava.
- She left Scutari in a French vessel for Marseilles under an assumed name (to avoid publicity).
- May 1910 was the Jubilee of the founding of the Nightingale Training School in New York. There were then over one thousand training schools for nurses in the United States alone.

# CHAPTER 15

# Letters

## A TRIP TO EGYPT

39 letters written to her family, on her return her sister Parthenope insisted on putting her letters into print, Florence refused—Nevertheless Parthe persisted and if it had not been for Parthe—these letters would have been lost to us.

> In one of her letters to her father Florence tells him that she is desperate to escape the bitterness and pain of women—
>
> "Why cannot a woman follow abstractions like a man? Has she less imagination, less intellect, less self-devotion, less religion than a man? I think not."

Perhaps no one in the world ever understood Florence Nightingale better than her father. When in 1861 the death of Sidney Herbert reduced her to the blackest despair, he wrote—

"My hand and heart misgive at the thought of approaching within the shadow of such grief as yours. Perhaps, it is better to magnify it not to try to soften."

**Feb 19, 1855**
Florence wrote to Sidney Herbert—
"The last few days have made a marked improvement in the health of the patients'—whereas in the first days of February we buried 506 from the hospitals at Scutari alone, on the ninth day 72—during the last 24 hours, we have lost only 10 (out of twenty one hundred in this [i.e., Barrack hospital]) only thirty (out of the whole of hospitals of the Bosphorus). It is not much more than ½%.
Nightingale strongly believed that the Army needed reforms—both in peace and in war—She requested the Queen to give her a royal commission to look into the state of the army. This was finally granted—

**John Sutherland wrote to Florence Nightingale:**
"I am led to believe that there must be a foundation of truth under the old myth about the Amazon women somewhere in the East of Scutari. All I can say is that if you had been queen of that respectable body in old days, Alexander the Great, would have had rather a bad chance." (John Sutherland Commissioner Royal Commission).

In early January 1874, sometime after 3.30 AM—Wen, Florence's father had a stroke which proved to be fatal no one was beside him except his valet.

**Letter written to Parthe (Florence's sister)**
"I do not think his death awful for him, he was the purest mind and I think the most single heart I have ever known. It is his New Year; he was quite ready to part with his life. He always wished to go out of the world quietly."

November 29, 1855 wrote Fanny Nightingale to her daughter at Scutari.

"This 29th November, the most interesting day in thy mother's life. It is very late my child, but I cannot go to bed without telling you that your meeting has been a glorious one. I believe that you will be more indifferent than any of us to your fame, but be glad that we feel this is a proud day for us; for the like has never happened before, but will, I trust, from your example, gladden the hearts of many future mothers."

**I work in the wards all day and write all night.**
There were no night nurses, but Florence Nightingale, lamp in hand, each night traversed alone the four miles of beds it was generally far into the night before she again reached her quarter not to rest but to write reports, and also letters for the soldiers and relatives of dead soldiers.

A letter written to Dr. Bowman November 15, 1854, Florence Nightingale gives definite statistics:

"_____ on Thursday last (i.e., November 8) we had 1715 sick and wounded in the hospital (among whom, 120 cholera patients) and 650 severely wounded in _____ the General Hospital _____ when a message came to me to prepare for 500 wounded."

She held the Army in high esteem, she wrote before I came here—I have never seen so teachable and helpful a class as the Army generally.

- Give them opportunity promptly and securely to send money home and they will use it.

## Chapter 15: Letters

- Give then a school and a lecture and they will come to it.
- Give them a book and a game and a magic Lanthorn and they will lay off drinking.
- Give them suffering and they will bear it.
- Give them work and they will do it.

I had rather have to do with the Army generally than with any other class I have ever attempted to serve.

> "No one can feel for the Army as I do" [1857]

Florence Nightingale, letter to Thomas Longmore on the Geneva Convention (23rd July, 1864).

"I need hardly say that I think its views most absurd—just such as would originate in a little state like Geneva, which never can see war. They tend to remove responsibility from Governments. They are practically impracticable. And voluntary effort is desirable, just in so far as it can be incorporated into the military system. If the present regulations are not sufficient to provide for the wounded they should be made so. But it would be an error to revert to a voluntary system, or to weaken the military character of the present system by introducing voluntary effort, unless such efforts were to become military in its organization."

She was not exaggerating when she wrote to the Herberts on July 11, 1855.

"Now, I will say what I would not except under this pressure, and what I would not, if you were in office have said—what I will never say to anyone else. We pulled this hospital through for 4 months and without us, it would have come to a stand still".

Florence Nightingale's, letter published in the English woman's Review (January, 1869).

"I have no peculiar gifts. And I can honestly assure any young lady, if she will but try to walk, she will soon be able to run the "appointed course". But then she must first learn to walk, and so when she runs she must run with patience. (Most people don't even try to walk). But I would also say to all young ladies who are called to any particular vocation, qualify yourself for it as a man does for his work. Don't think you can undertake it otherwise".

The appalling conditions at Scutari
April 1855 letter to Benjamin Hawes.

"Forty women, living closely packed in narrow quarters under new discipline and in a Barrack—women too whose tempers and habits are unknown present great obstacles to management."

Unshrinking Heroism
Nov. 14 wrote to Dr Bowman.

"In the midst of this appalling horror (we are steeped up to our necks in blood)—there is good..... As I went my night rounds among the newly wounded that first night, there was not one murmur, not are groan, the strict discipline, the most absolute silence and quiet prevailed, only the step of the sentry, and I heard one man say, I was dreaming of my friends at home and another said and I was thinking of them.

These poor fellows bear pain and mutilation with unshrinking heroism, and die or are cut up without a complaint. Not so the officers, but we have nothing to do with the officers."

Florence Nightingale spent as many hours a day as she could on individual patient care. On the days when hundreds of new patient's were disembarked from the transport ships, she was the nurse who worked the longest hours and was one of the most effective.

"Her nerve in wonderful, I have been with her at very severe operations; she was more than equal to the trial. She has an utter disregard of contagion; I have known her spend hours over men dying of cholera or fever. The more awful in every sense any particular case, especially if it was that of a dying man, her slight form would be seen bending over him, administering to his ease in every way in her power, and seldom quitting his side till death released him." Osborne

> As a Chaplin, Osborne had full access to the wards at Scutari.

**NOTE**
Traveling gentlemen like:
Rev. the Hon Sidney Godolphin Osborne a good friend of Sidney Herbert, was a doctor, an Anglican minister, and a writer for the Times.

December 31, 1852. She wrote in her diary:

"I am so glad this year is over, nevertheless it has not been wasted I trust _____ I have remodeled my whole religious belief _____ All my admirers are married _____ and I stand with all the world before me _____ It has been a baptism of fire this year."

# CHAPTER 16

# We Know Now, What Was Not Known Then

We know now, what was not known then, but was advocated and implemented by Florence Nightingale.
- That typhus is spread by body lice.
- That fleas rats and flies are key vectors of disease.
- That good nutrition is specially important to the sick.
- That dysentery, diarrhea and fever can often be caused by improperly prepared food.
- That a wound not cleaned and debrided of necrotic tissue everyday will develop gangrene.
- That Vitamin C is essential to the formation of scar tissue.
- That morale has an important bearing on the human immune system.

> The care and attention given by her, also her night rounds, raised the general morale and also helped to identify and detect diseases in their early stage.

- That a therapeutic environment is congenial to recovery (which she established in the Barrack hospitals)—
  - Good ventilation in the wards.
  - Hygienic measures is a must and basic to prevent infection and to promote recovery.
  - Fresh air.
  - Clean laundry (set up a laundry).
  - Regular change of patients personal clothing.
  - Cleanliness of the skin.
  - Use of separate sponge cloth for each patient.
  - Therapeutic diet (set up a special kitchen) was particularly regarding the serving of cooking, soft diet which was easily digestible.
  - Spacing between beds.

- Providing of privacy—provided screens specially during procedures.
- Practiced advocacy and protected the soldiers rights.
- Made provision for recreation.
- Conducted educational programs.
- Initiated a Remittance Scheme (wherein soldiers could send part of their savings home to the families).
- Practiced holistic-transpersonal caring.

Today we teach and stress on the importance of critical thinking skills. In 1873, Florence Nightingale developed a model for independent nursing schools to teach *Critical Thinking, Attention to Patient's Individual Needs, and Respect for Patient's Rights.*

- Introduced the concept of care plans and stressed on holistic nursing.
- Brought professionalism into nursing—always put patient safety and welfare first.
- She used statistics to understand and to make others aware of patient care.
- She mentioned and reported systematically outcomes of care.
- She believed and implemented with great success—total patient care.
- Developed a hospital statistical system for comparison of:
  - Outcomes of care
  - Mortality
  - Morbidity
- She had a vision of what nursing should be and established it as a scientific modern profession.

# CHAPTER 17

# Nurses Corner

Florence Nightingale was ever ready to impart practical advice and share her experiences with all who needed them. She campaigned tirelessly to improve health standards.

These Alphabets of nursing have been written, keeping in mind the nursing virtues which all nurses must cultivate and adorn; an interesting feature is that each virtue has been high-lighted by demonstrating anecdotes and situations from the life of Florence Nightingale. I hope it will help each nurse to commit herself/himself to quality.

The 'Nurses Corner' has two sections:
  Section—A   Alphabets of Nursing
  Section—B   International Nurses Day Themes from 1988-2008

## SECTION A

### ALPHABETS OF NURSING

The intuitive mind is a sacred gift and the rational mind is a faithful servant. We have created a society that honors the servant and has forgotten the gift.

**Albert Einstein**

**Chapter 17:** Nurses Corner

> For us who nurse, our Nursing is a thing, which, unless in it we are making progress every year, every month, every week, take my word for it, we are going back.
>
> **Florence Nightingale**

**Chapter 17:** Nurses Corner

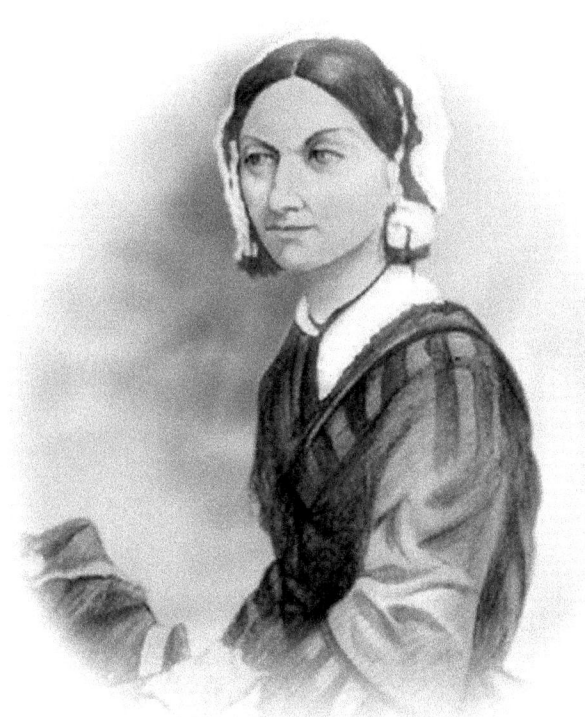

**Born May 12, 1820
Died August 13, 1910**

## Chapter 17: Nurses Corner

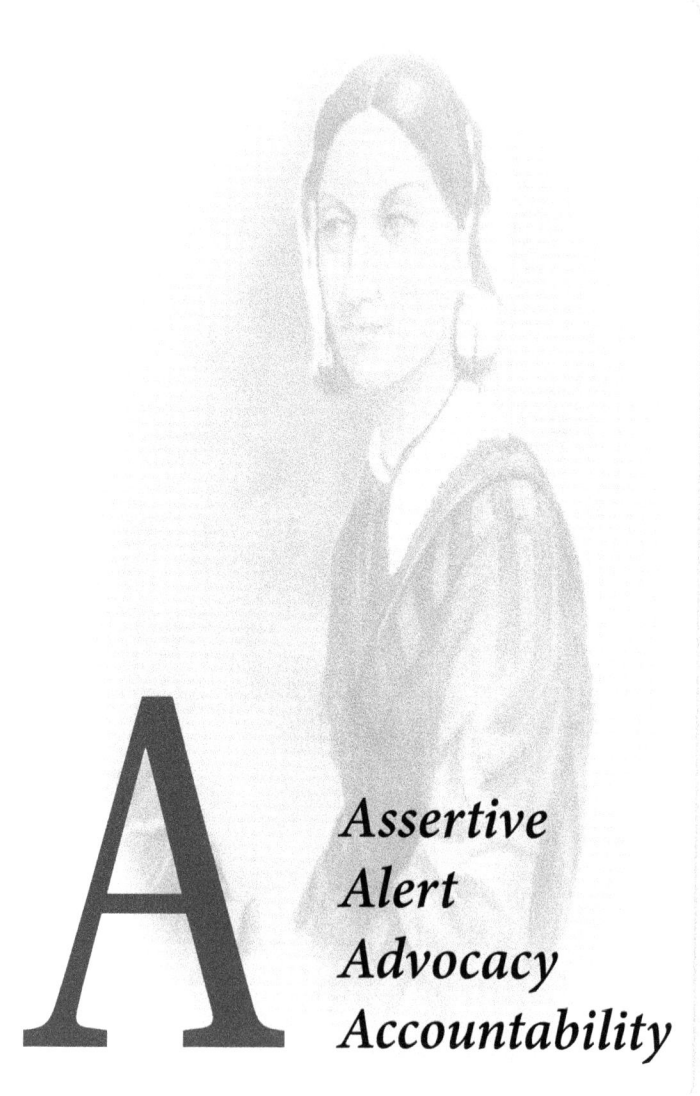

**A** *Assertive*
*Alert*
*Advocacy*
*Accountability*

## Chapter 17: Nurses Corner

*"I stand at the altar of the murdered men, & while I live, I fight their cause"* (1856)

*Florence Nightingale*

**On Her Return From Crimea**

- She felt that something constructive must be done to ameliorate future army conditions while public opinion was still keenly alive to all defects. She wasted no time, and within 3 months from her return was deep in official work.
- "We can do no more for those who have suffered and died in their country's service; they need our help no longer; their spirits are with God who gave them. It remains to us to strive that their sufferings may not have been endured in vain—to endeavour so to learn from experience as to lessen such suffering in future by forethought and wise imagination."

*Florence Nightingale*

"Our aspirations are our possibilities."

*Robert Browning*

## Chapter 17: Nurses Corner

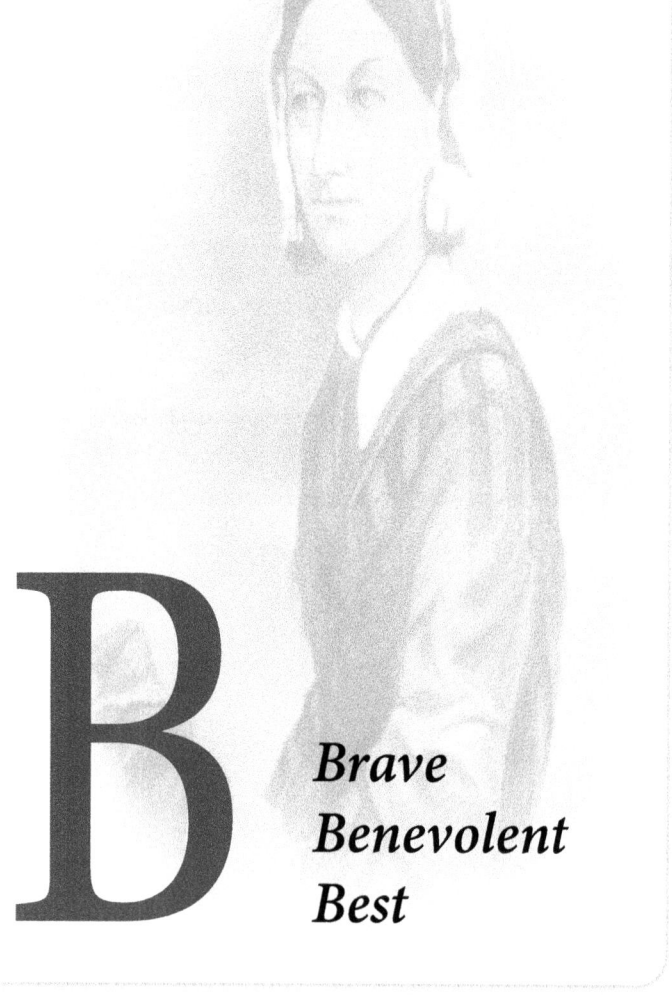

**B**
*Brave*
*Benevolent*
*Best*

## Chapter 17: Nurses Corner

*"I can stand out the war with any man."*
*Florence Nightingale*

- She justified this statement. She courageously withstood the grisly sights and horrors of war.
  Wherever there was the worst suffering, there she would appear as if by magic, to hold a hand, to soothe, and to infuse the victim with courage to endure and to hope.
- Florence Nightingale was an outstanding nurse. She was ready to dress the most appalling wounds or stuff lint into a spurting artery until a surgeon appeared. She was undeterred by the terrible physical deformities of the wounded.

**"Courage is fear that has said its prayers."**
**Italian Proverb**

**"How very little can be done under the spirit of fear."**
**Florence Nightingale**

## Chapter 17: Nurses Corner

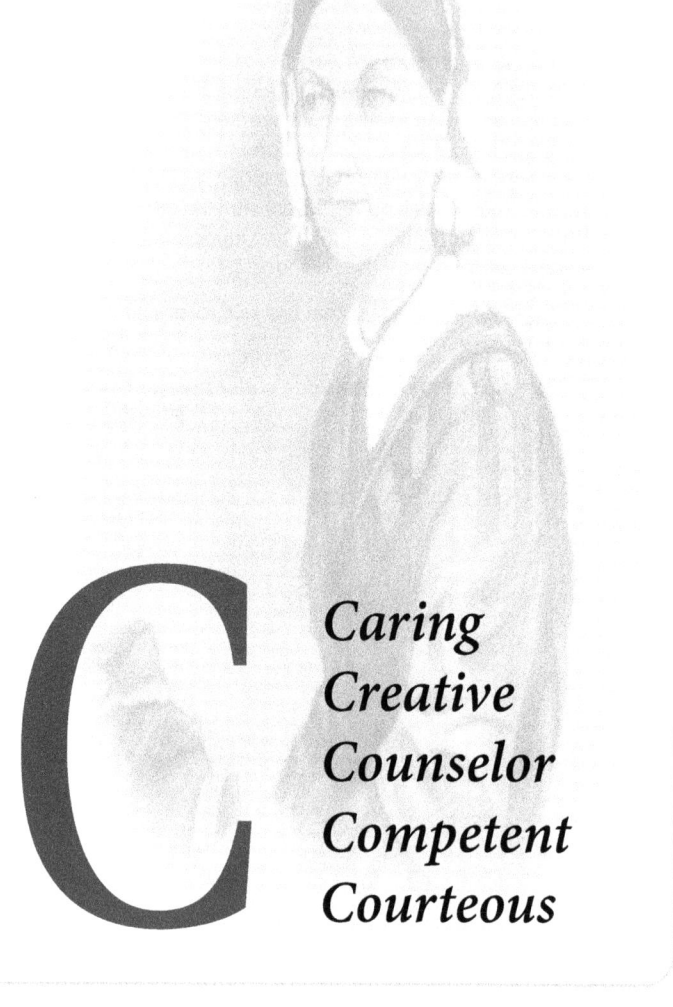

**C** *Caring*
*Creative*
*Counselor*
*Competent*
*Courteous*

## Chapter 17: Nurses Corner

*"Everyone likes a caring person in their life."*

- "All the results of good nursing .... may be ..... negatived by one defect, viz ...... by not knowing how to manage that what you do when you are there, shall be done when you are not there".
- Florence Nightingale liked to do massage, a comforting therapeutic technique; she would bring water, tea and jelly, she would wash parts of man's body in an attempt to make him more comfortable, she would change a sheet, or a shirt, wipe away sweat, and supply that comfortable old staple of British home life, a hot water bottle. Much of what she did was psychological, and here none of her nurses could come close to her. She talked to the men, listened to them, and specially for the dying wrote letters.
- What a confidential nurse should be "And remember every nurse should be one who is to be depended upon, in other words, capable of being a confidential nurse—she must be no gossip, no vain talker".

**Florence Nightingale**

"It's not how much you say but how much you care that brings the most comfort."

"Caring is active prayer."

## Chapter 17: Nurses Corner

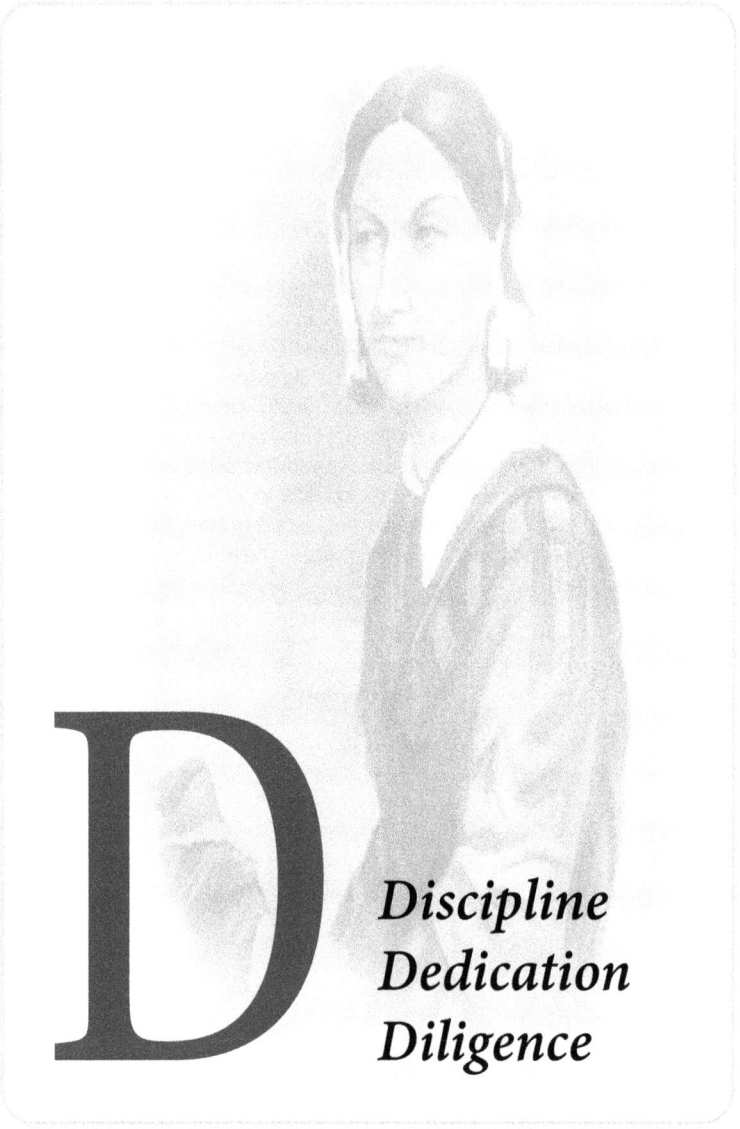

**D**
*Discipline*
*Dedication*
*Diligence*

## Chapter 17: Nurses Corner

*"A wise child loves discipline."*

*Proverbs 13:1*

- Nursing without discrimination "The sect of the Good Samaritan 'She belongs to a sect which unfortunately is a very rare one the sect of the Good Samaritan' (Said of Florence Nightingale):
- "True caring does not discriminate based on race, religion, age, behavior, or any other characteristic. This is one of the challenges of being a professional nurse".

**"You need endurance and discipline to win a race."**

## Chapter 17: Nurses Corner

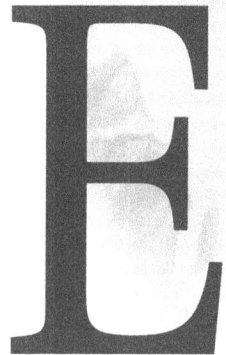

**E**
*Excellence*
*Efficient*
*Educator*
*Economical*
*Evaluator*

## Chapter 17: Nurses Corner

*"No one can feel for the army as I do." (1857)*
*Florence Nightingale*

- "Florence Nightingale held the Army in high esteem. She wrote: "before I came here (Scutari)—I have never seen so teachable and helpful a class as the Army; I had rather have to do with Army generally than any other class I have ever attempted to serve".
- "The everyday management of a large ward, let alone of a hospital—the knowing what are the laws of life and death for men, and what the laws of health for wards (and wards are healthy or unhealthy, mainly according to the knowledge or ignorance of the nurse)—are not these matter of sufficient importance and difficulty to require learning by experience and careful inquiring, just as much as any other art?."

**Florence Nightingale**

"Let each founder train as many in her/his spirit as he/she can. Their pupils will in their turn be founder also."

**Florence Nightingale**

"Strive for excellence rather than perfection."

## Chapter 17: Nurses Corner

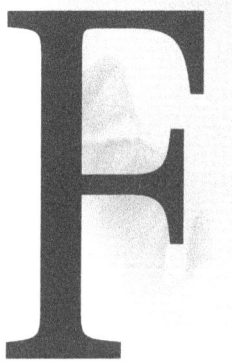

**F** *Far-sighted*
*Firm*
*Friendly*
*Focused*

## Chapter 17: Nurses Corner

*"Florence Nightingale was patient-focused and patient-need focused."*

- February 22, 1855: She floated a new scheme—to set-up a medical school in an abandoned kiosk on the esplanade above the Barrack Hospital.
  She planned to fund the building for occupancy out of her own pocket—Doctors would then be called from England armed with their own scientific instruments, and would teach and also do research.
- Florence Nightingale was a Unitarian. The Unitarians believe that mankind has the power to continuously improve itself by observation and the use of reason.
- Farsightedness—[Attending to Scientific Needs]. She took a house at her own expense to serve as a dissecting room and fitted it up with instruments also for the use of the army doctors. This small experiment was destined to be the nuclear of the Army Medical School.

**Florence Nightingale saw in Scutari: "The finest opportunity for advancing the cause of medicine and exacting it into a science".**

**"When you are intensely focused you are pursuing your conscious mind."**

**Chapter 17:** Nurses Corner

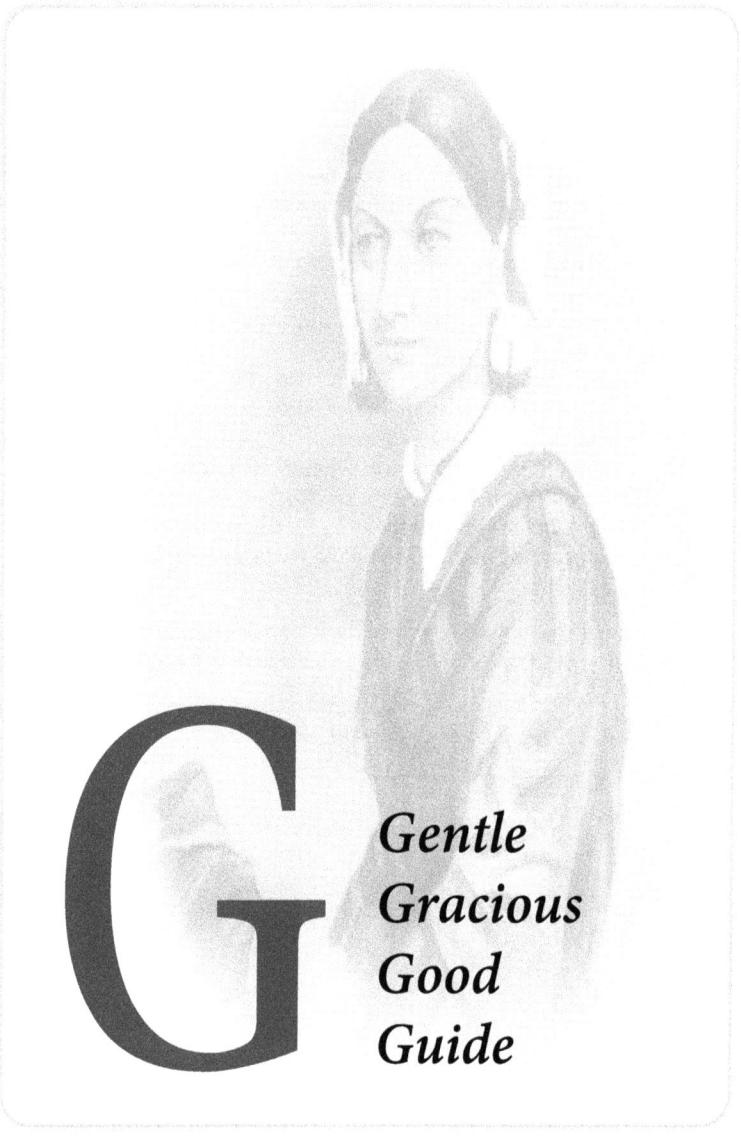

# G
*Gentle*
*Gracious*
*Good*
*Guide*

## Chapter 17: Nurses Corner

*"Goodness is the only investment that never fails."*

- ❑ **"Gentle caring**—When the wounded and sick were brought to the hospital—She would mobilize her nurses to wash the men, feed them regular, digestible, nutritious food, and gave them clean clothes, clean sheets and blankets and reasonably comfortable beds."
- ❑ **"Gentle presence**—What a comfort to see her pass. She would speak to one, nod and smile to as many more; but she could not do it to all you know. We lay there by the hundreds, but we could kiss her shadow as it fell and lay our heads on the pillow again content."

**Anonymous**

**People will remember what you achieve—
not what you promised to achieve.**

- ❑ True caring emphasizes the nurses' enabling presence.
- ❑ Nursing is to be a healing presence in people's lives.

**Chapter 17:** Nurses Corner

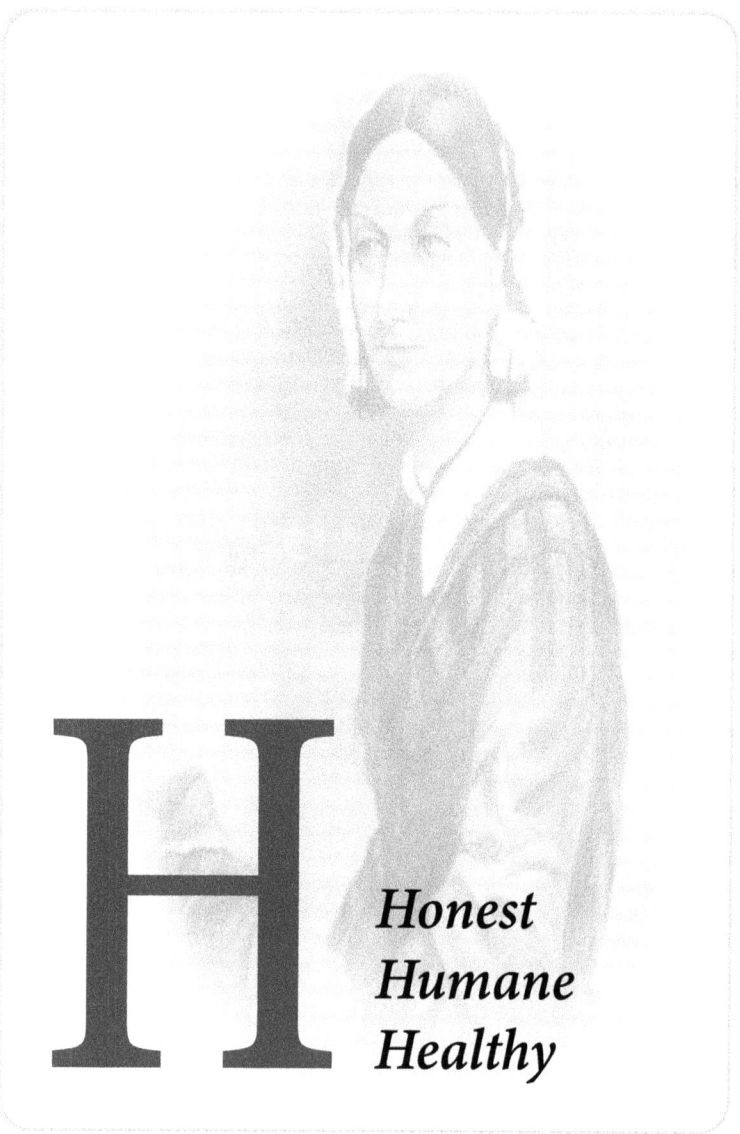

# H
## *Honest*
## *Humane*
## *Healthy*

*"The head cannot reach higher than does the heart."*
Orison Swett Marden

**Advice to Nursing Students 1873**

- "The honour does not lie in putting on Nursing like your uniform. Honour lies in loving perfection, consistency, and in working hard for it: in being ready to work patiently; ready to say not "How clever I am" but "I am not yet worthy; and I will live to deserve to be called a Trained Nurse." Florence Nightingale
- **The White Heart**—The white heart is the universal symbol for nursing. It is meant to characterize the caring, knowledge and humanity that infuse the work and spirit of nursing. The white heart is also a unifying symbol for nurses globally.

  White was selected because it brings together all colors, demonstrating nursing's acceptance of all people. White also has a worldwide association with nursing, caring, hygiene and comfort. The heart shape communicates humanity and the central place that nursing has in quality health care.

"A heart that cares is a happy heart."
Italian Proverb

## Chapter 17: Nurses Corner

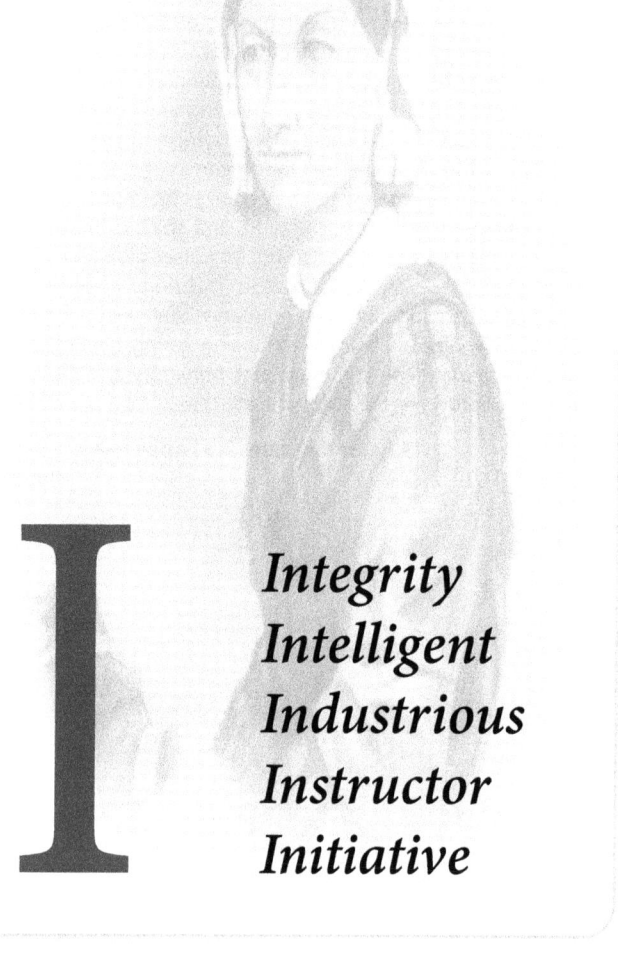

**I**
*Integrity*
*Intelligent*
*Industrious*
*Instructor*
*Initiative*

## Chapter 17: Nurses Corner

*"Integrity—There is no legacy as rich as integrity."*

- "It is said that she did an enormous amount of work which big and strong men were unable to do. She used to work nearly twenty hours, day and night. When the women working under her went to sleep, she, lamp in hand, went out alone at midnight to the patient's bed-side, comforted them, and herself gave them whatever food and other things were necessary."

(Extract from Mahatma Gandhi's article on Florence Nightingale published in Indian Opinion, September 9, 1915)

**"Imagination is more important than knowledge."**
**Albert Einstein**

Chapter 17: Nurses Corner

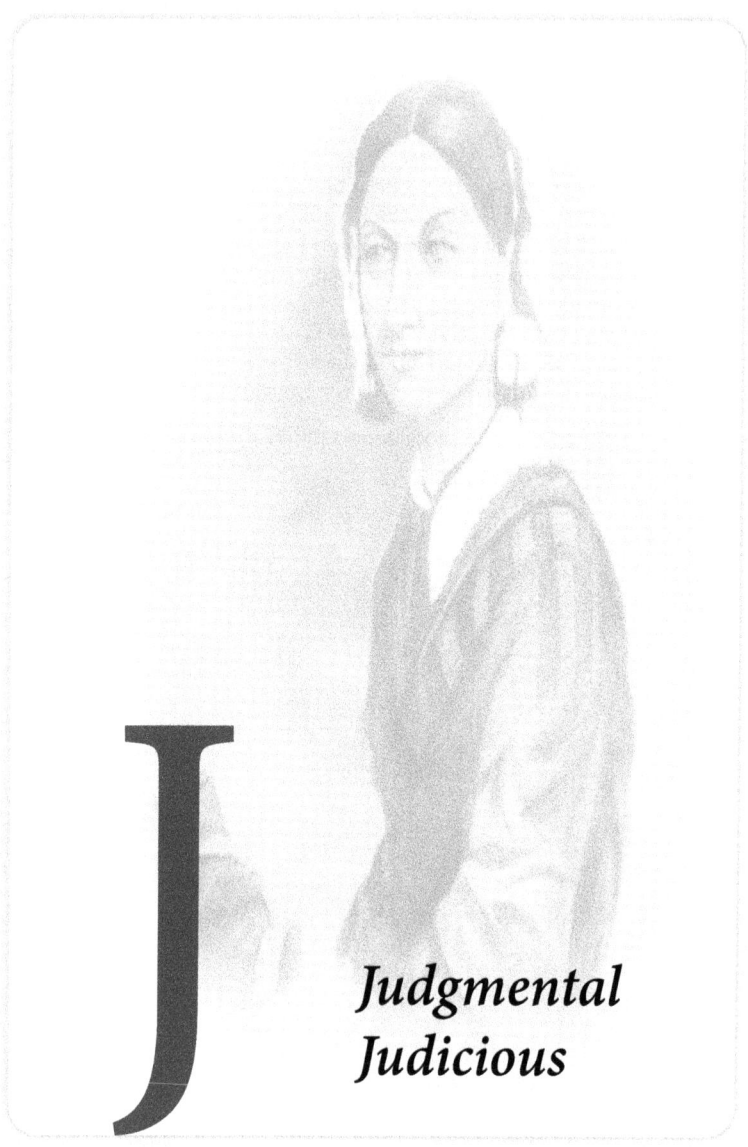

# J
**Judgmental
Judicious**

## Chapter 17: Nurses Corner

*"We cannot direct the wind —
But we can adjust the sails."*

- "Florence Nightingale faced gender related frustrations but on the wards remained calm, quiet and polite (whatever the provocation) she never raised her voice and acted discreetly according to the situation."

    **"Be just and fear not."**
    **William Shakespeare**

**Chapter 17:** Nurses Corner

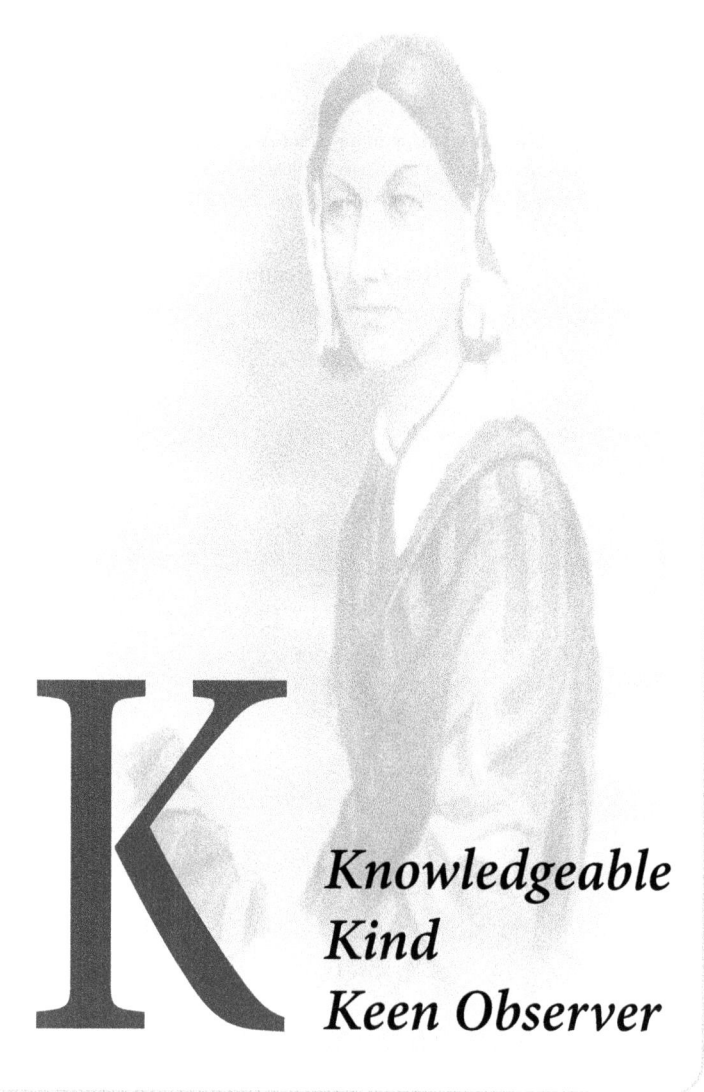

**K** *Knowledgeable*
*Kind*
*Keen Observer*

*"Nothing can be accomplished until you begin."*
*Ira Hayes*

- In pursuit of knowledge Florence Nightingale was remorseless. She was brilliant, she was focused, she was competitive, and she identified learning, correctly, as an avenue of power.

  **"Every addition to true knowledge is an addition to human power"**
  **Horace Mann**

  **"Even when I think what a human intellect may become by industry, ambition comes before me like 'Circe' with her cup to tempt me."**
  **Florence Nightingale**

**Chapter 17:** Nurses Corner

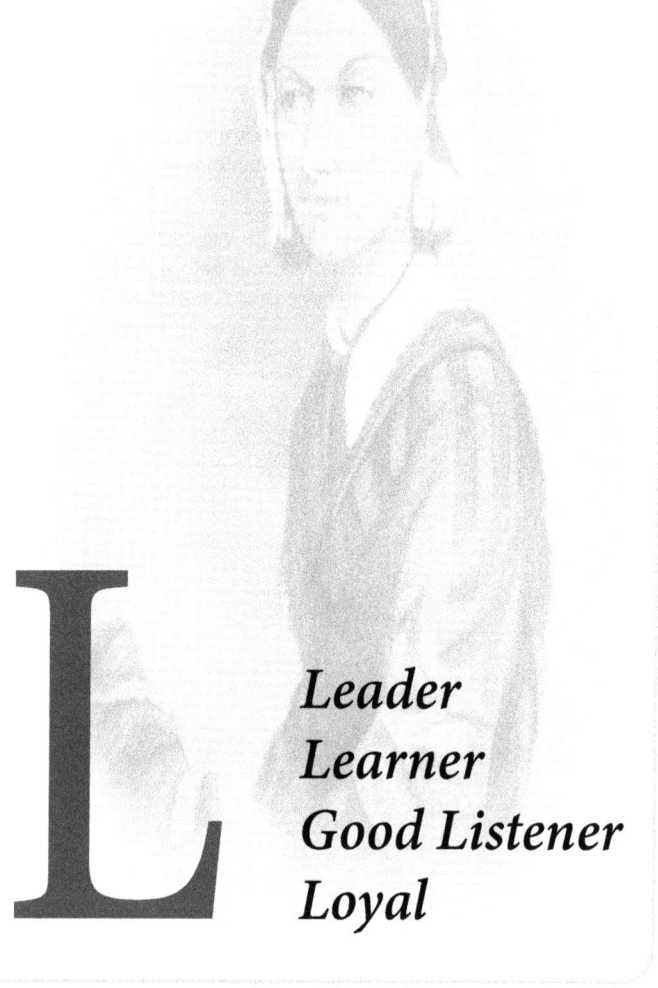

L

*Leader*
*Learner*
*Good Listener*
*Loyal*

*"Leadership is action, not position."*
Donald H Mc Gannan

**Life doesn't require us to make good; it asks only that we give our best at each level of experience.**
**Harold Ruopp**

- In her letters to Herbert, Florence allowed her anger and frustration to show—but on the wards, Florence Nightingale remained calm, cordial and polite whatever the provocation, and was famous among her nurses for never raising her voice. This combination of strategies was extremely effective, and Nightingale's capacity as a *leader* awed her friends and put the fear of God into her enemies."

### Good Listener

- Listening to patient's (joys and sorrows) is itself an art.
Henry David Thoreau
- "If you listen to your patient long enough he/she will tell you what is wrong with him/her."
- Talking to the patient means listening to a patient.

**"Learn to listen, listen to learn."**

**Chapter 17:** Nurses Corner

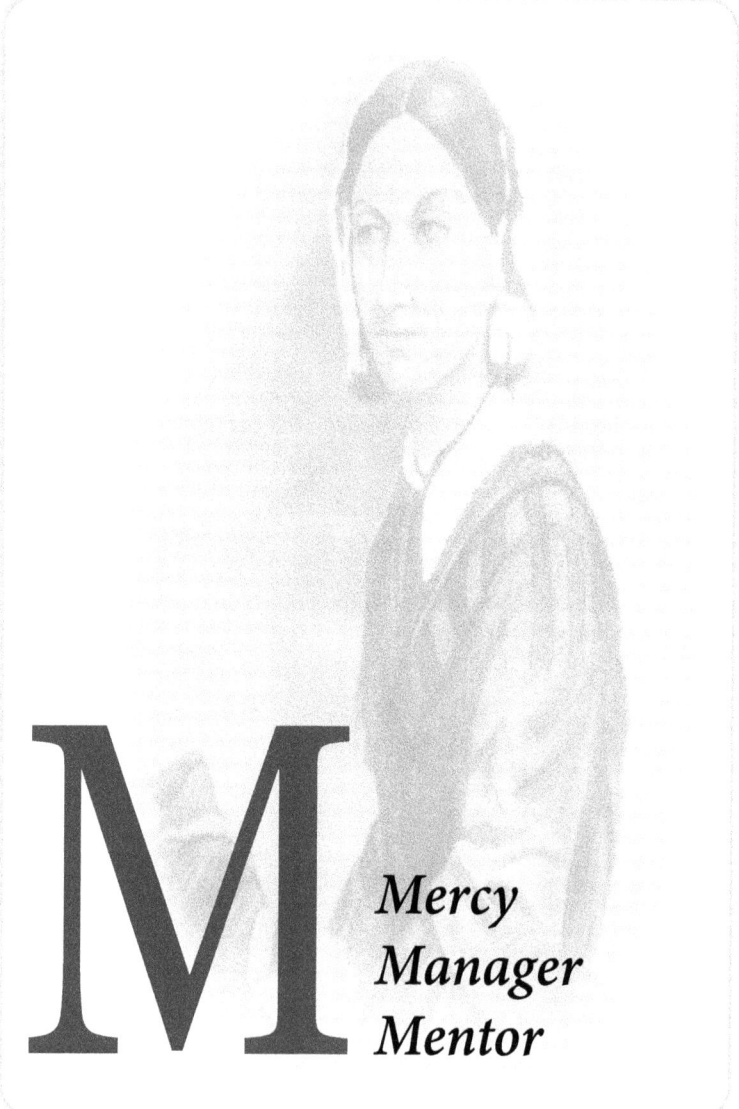

M *Mercy*
*Manager*
*Mentor*

*"Management is doing things right leadership is doing the right thing."*

Stephen R Covey (1989)

### Management Skills

- Scutari was lacking in the most basic elements needed to good nursing, but Florence Nightingale organized care and got practical things implemented fast. Nightingale embarked on a vigorous campaign to wash the men, feed them regular, digestible, nutritious food and give them clean clothes, clean sheets and blankets and reasonably comfortable beds.
- "Nursing encompasses autonomous and collaborative care of individuals of all ages, families, groups and communities, sick or well and in all settings. Nursing includes the promotion of health, prevention of illness, and the care of ill, disabled and dying people."
- Advocacy, promotion of a safe environment, research, participation in shaping health policy and in patient and health systems management, and education are also key nursing roles.
- Merciful "One day Florence saw same boys tormenting a tiny owl that had fallen from the nest. She bought the owl from the children and christened it Athena."

**"All of life is the management of risk, not its elimination."**

**Walter Wriston**

**Chapter 17:** Nurses Corner

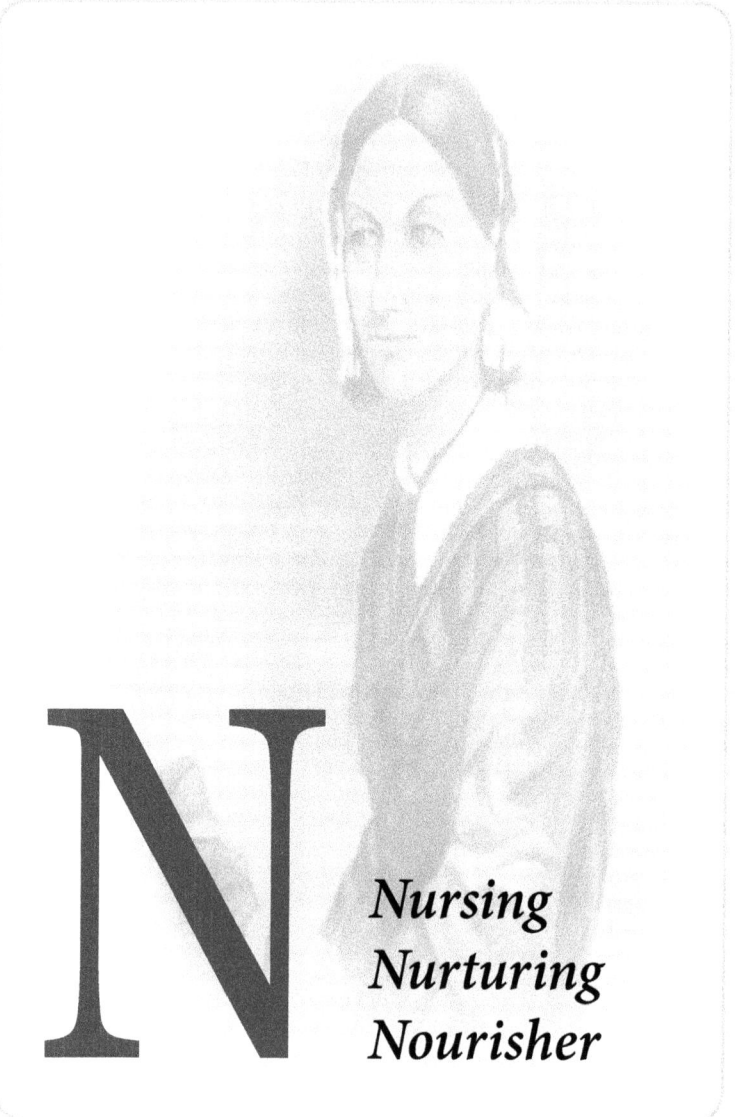

# N
*Nursing*
*Nurturing*
*Nourisher*

## Chapter 17: Nurses Corner

*"Florence believed: To nurse was also to hold a hand, to look with love; to be there for the dying."*

- For at least half of her twenty one months in Turkey and Crimea, Nightingale spent as many hours a day as she could on individual patient care.
- "Nightingale was famous among the medical staff for appearing when least expected and most needed."
- Osborne: "Her nerve is wonderful; I have been with her at very severe operations; she was more than equal to the trial. She has an utter disregard of contagion; I have known her spend hours over men dying of cholera or fever. The more awful in every sense any particular case, specially if it was that of a dying man, her slight form would be seen bending over him, administering to his ease in every way in her power, and seldom, quitting his side till death released him."

*"Nursing is nurturing, caring for and about people."*

## Chapter 17: Nurses Corner

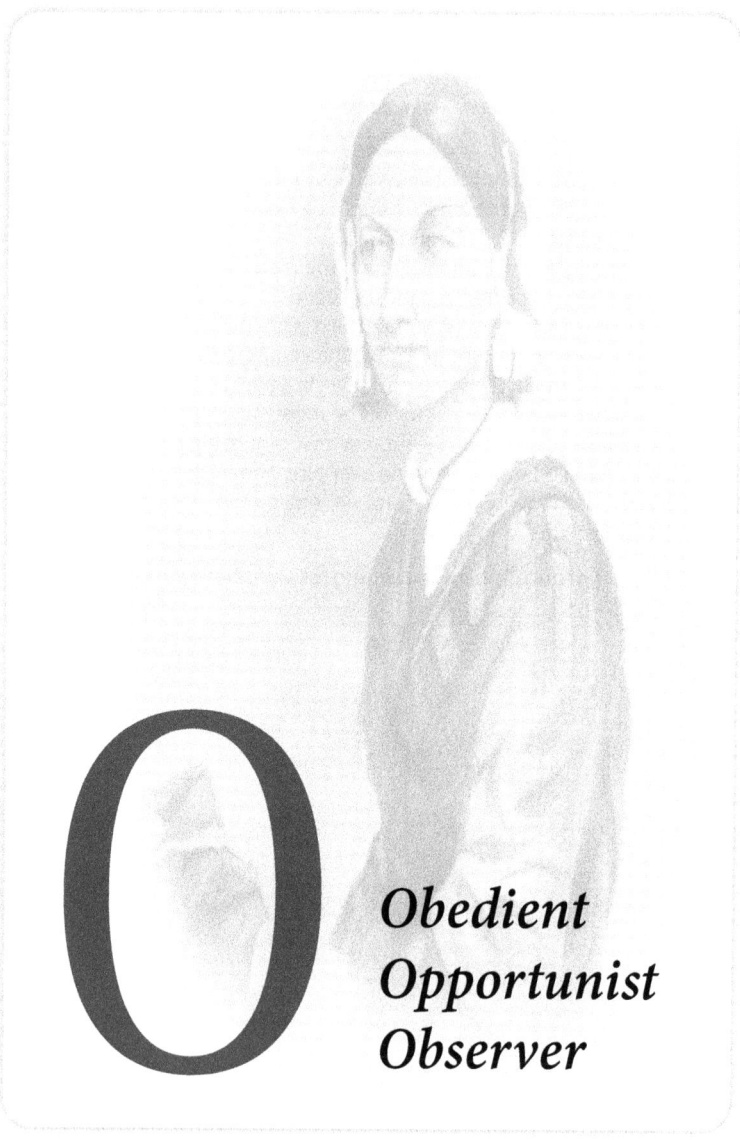

# O
*Obedient*
*Opportunist*
*Observer*

## Chapter 17: Nurses Corner

*"There is, unquestionably, physiognomy of disease.
Let the nurse learn it."*

***Florence Nightingale***

- ❏ But if you cannot get the habit of observation one way or another you had better give up being a nurse, for it is not your calling, however kind and anxious you may be.

  Florence Nightingale

- ❏ Keen Observation in Nursing—In dwelling upon the vital importance of sound observation, it must never be lost sight of what observation is for. It is not for the sake of piling up miscellaneous information or curious facts, but for the sake of saving life and increasing health and comfort.

  Florence Nightingale

**"Nursing is 90% observation."**

# Chapter 17: Nurses Corner

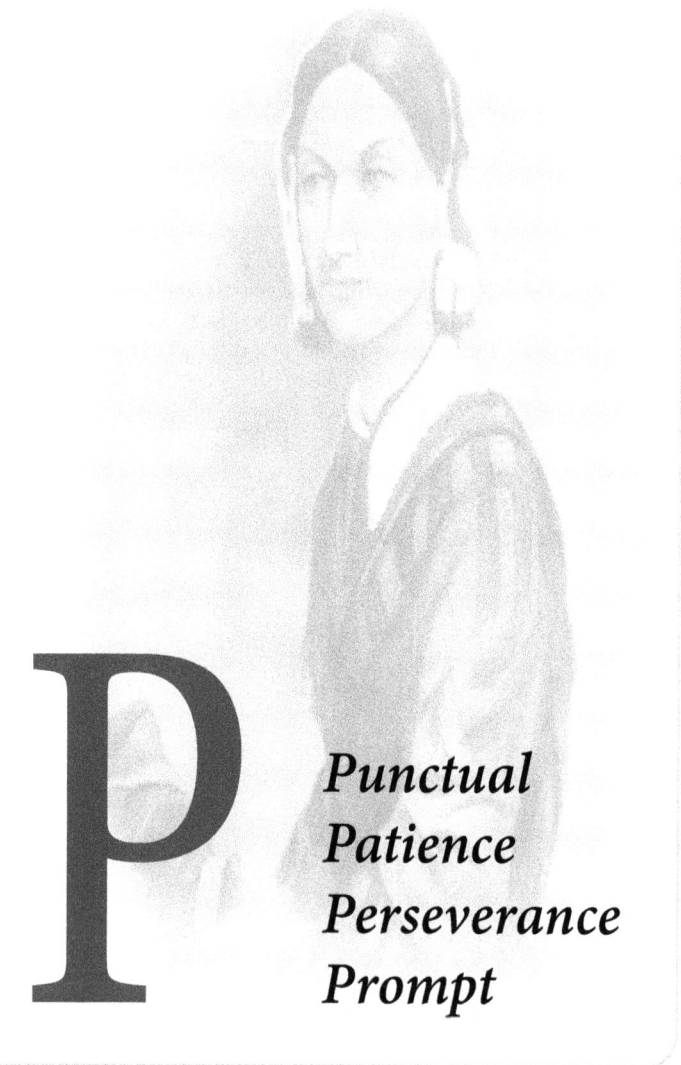

# P
*Punctual*
*Patience*
*Perseverance*
*Prompt*

## Chapter 17: Nurses Corner

> *"Ingenuity and perseverance (and these really constitute the good nurse) might save more lives than we wot of."*
>
> ***Florence Nightingale***

- "For us who nurse, our Nursing is a thing, which, unless in it we are making progress every year, every month, every week, take my word for it, we are going back."

  Florence Nightingale

- 'Let whoever is In-charge keep this simple question in her head (not how can I always do this right thing myself) but how can I provide for this right thing to always be done'.

  Florence Nightingale

- **"Patience, perseverance and focused, planned learning:** Florence Nightingale's letter published (January, 1869) "I have no peculiar gifts and I can honestly assure any young lady, if she will but try to walk, she will soon be able to run the 'appointed course', But then she must first learn to walk, and so when she runs, she must run with patience (Most people don't even try to walk). But I would also say to all young ladies who are called to any particular vocation, qualify yourself for it as a man does for his work. Don't think you can undertake it otherwise."

**"Professionals are those who do their
best even when they do not feel like it."**

**Chapter 17:** Nurses Corner

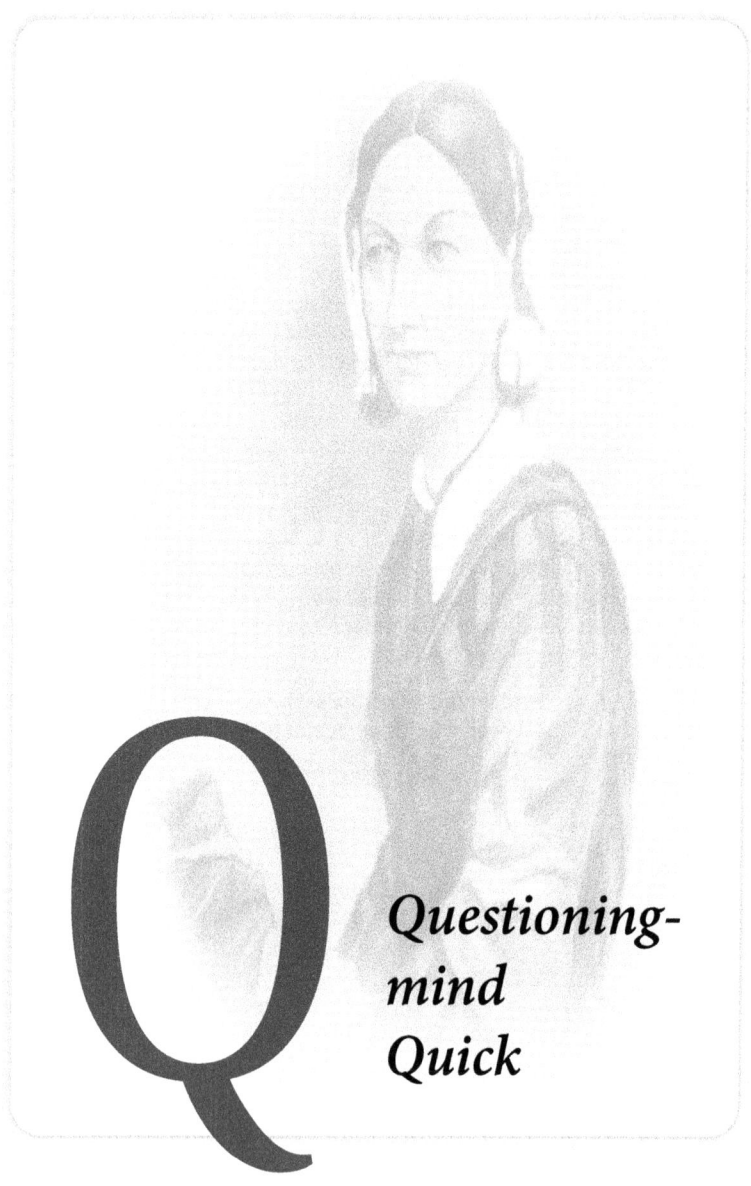

Q Questioning-
mind
Quick

## Chapter 17: Nurses Corner

*"The race for quality has no finish line."*

### Quality Care

- Florence Nightingale was an excellent bedsides nurse. She was quick to identify the needs of the patients and render quality care as and when required.

*"Quick to listen, slow to speak."*

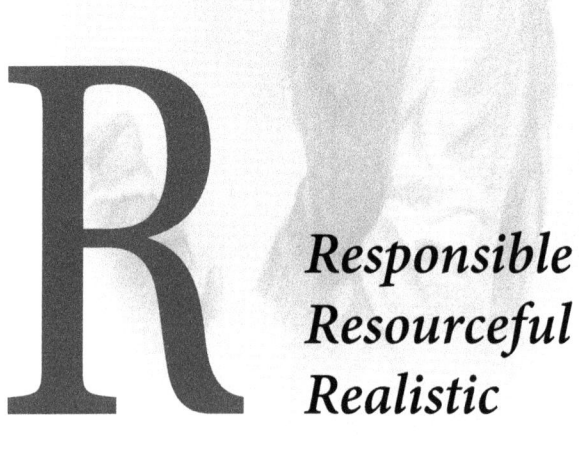

# R
*Responsible*
*Resourceful*
*Realistic*

"*It may seem a strange principle to enunciate as the very first requirement in a Hospital that it should do the sick no harm.*"

*Florence Nightingale*

### Responsible Caring

- "God lays down certain physical laws. Upon this carrying out such laws depends our responsibility (that much abused word), for how could we have any responsibility for actions, the results of which we could not foresee—which would be the case if the carrying out of his laws were not certain; yet we seem to be continually expecting that He will work a miracle—i.e., break His own laws expressly to relieve us of responsibility."

Florence Nightingale

**"Be responsible for your own conduct."**

## Chapter 17: Nurses Corner

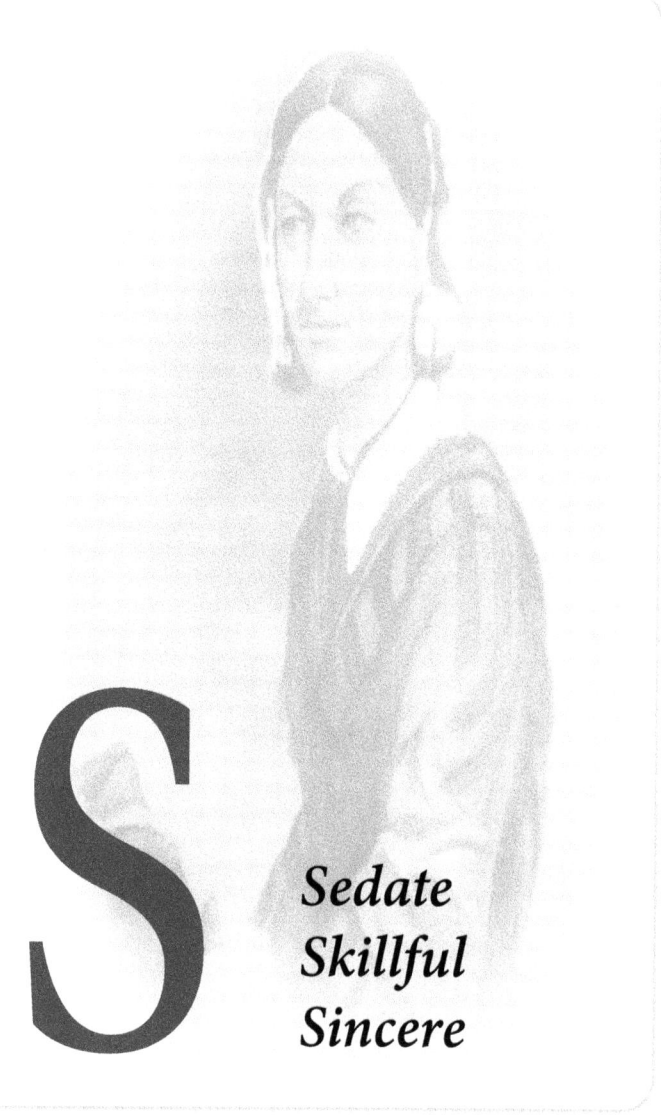

# S
*Sedate*
*Skillful*
*Sincere*

## Chapter 17: Nurses Corner

*"Sincerity is the strongest force in the world."*

Florence Nightingale—believed that morale has an important bearing on the human immune system.

She was a skilled bedside nurse and could assess and analyze the patient's needs—She was very particular regarding the patient's environment and she planned her care accordingly keeping in mind the therapeutic environment of the patient thus promoting healing—She kept the interest of her patient's in the forefront and provided care and that too with scanty resources. Yet she could bring down the mortality rate and render compassionate care to the wounded.

*"Search for better ways to do things and you will find success."*

*"The road to success is always under construction."*

- **S**  **S**incerity is the strongest force in the world
- **U**  Maximum **U**tilization of the ability you have spells success
- **C**  **C**ommit yourself to quality
- **C**  **C**hoose a goal, pursue it [stick to it]
- **E**  Make an **E**ducative moment of every failure
- **S**  **S**uccess is based on imagination, plus ambition and the will to work
- **S**  **S**uccess is a Journey

*"The only place 'success' comes before work is in the dictionary."*

**3 Things to Remember**
1. Your success helps many people, your failure helps no one.
2. "When you believe you can—you can!"
3. "There are no secrets to success.
   It is the result of:
   ➢ Preparation,
   ➢ Hard work, and
   ➢ Learning from failures."

**Chapter 17:** Nurses Corner

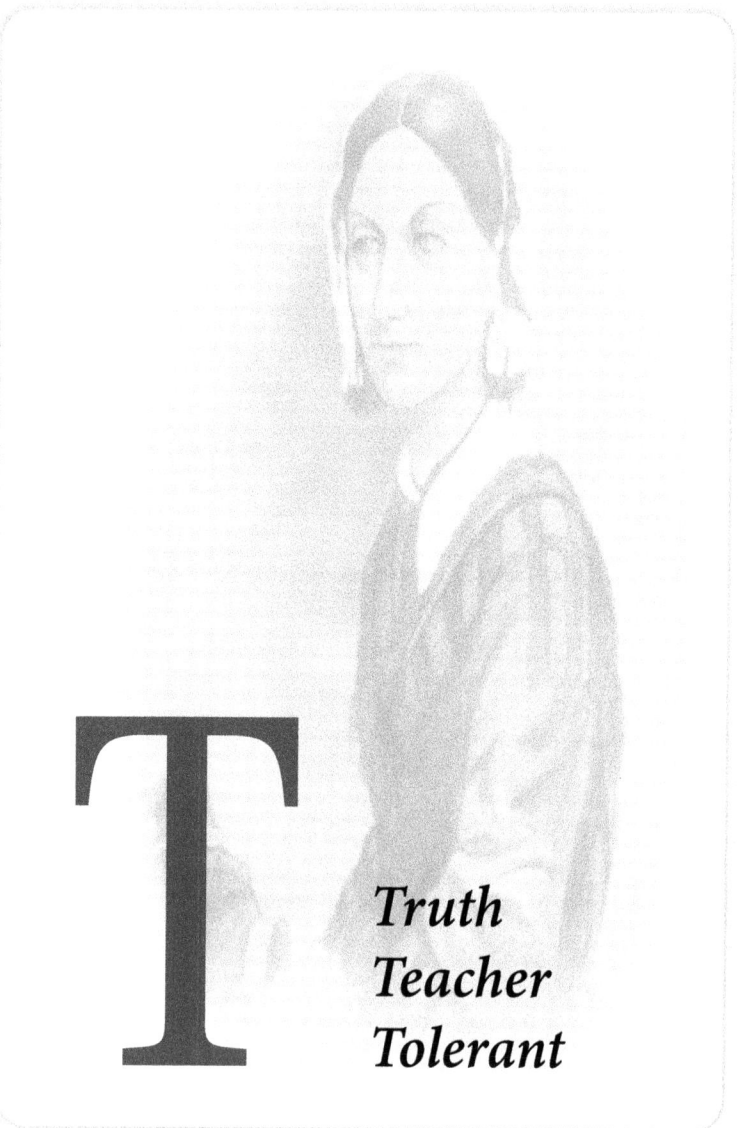

**T**

***Truth***
***Teacher***
***Tolerant***

## Chapter 17: Nurses Corner

*"The very first cannon of nursing was to keep the air as pure as possible."*

"Unnecessary noise, or noise that creates an expectation in the mind, is that which hurts the patient— All hurry and bustle is painful to the sick". Florence Nightingale

- "Always air your room, then from the outside air, if possible 'windows are made to open Doors are made to shut'—a truth which seems extremely difficult of apprehension."
  
  Florence Nightingale

- "Unnecessary noise, then is the most cruel absence of care which can be inflicted either on sick or well."
  
  Florence Nightingale

- "Without cleanliness, you cannot have all the effect of ventilation; without ventilation, you can have no thorough cleanliness."
  
  Florence Nightingale

- "Let us each and all realize the importance of on influence on others—stand shoulder to shoulder and not alone in a good cause."
  
  Florence Nightingale

**"Timing is the key to good judgment."**

# Chapter 17: Nurses Corner

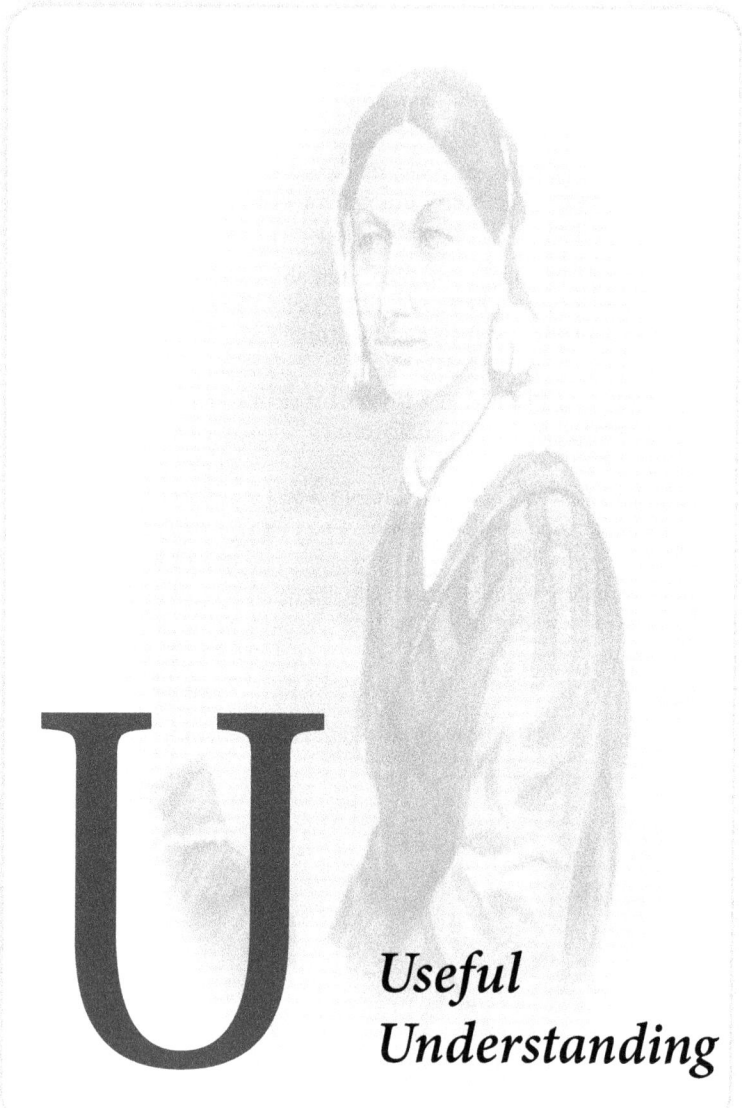

# U Useful Understanding

*"Life is about how you deal with adversity."*
*Diana Brooks*

Florence Nightingale had a deep understanding of human nature—she was an excellent bedside nurse with a strong power of observation and knew and assessed her patient's need and catered to their particular needs with compassion skill and understanding. When she went to Crimea—she made herself useful to all—specially the wounded she was like an 'Angel of Mercy' wherever there was the worst suffering there she would appear as if by magic to care for the sick—working from morning till night.

**"Hard work is the best investment a man can make."**
**Charles Schwab**

**"Those who undertake the work of aiding the sick and wounded must not be sentimental enthusiasts but downright lovers of hard work."**
**Florence Nightingale**

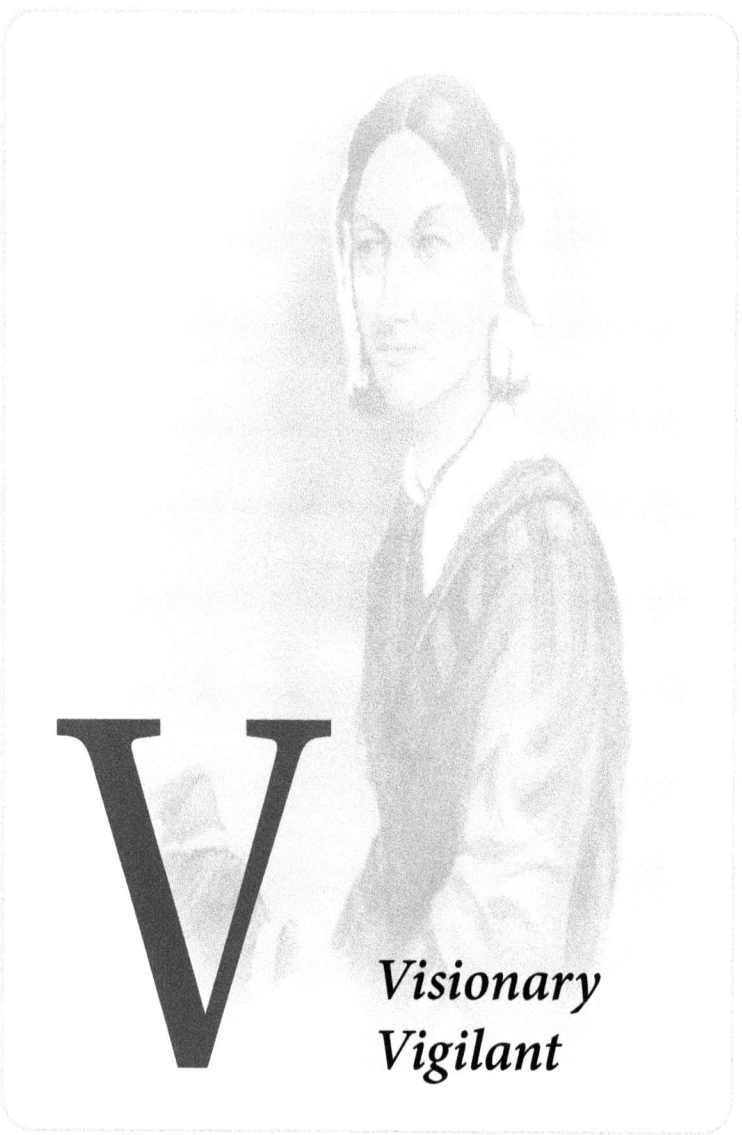

# V
*Visionary*
*Vigilant*

## Chapter 17: Nurses Corner

*"The only limits are, as always, those of vision."*

Jamas Broughten

**Vigilant**
- Constant vigilance and intelligent participation in all aspects of medical care.
- "Motivated orderlies and also doctors to be vigilant and alert, changing the 'inertia' that prevailed in all army hospitals."
- She rallied for systematic training but did not rate it higher than character—or imagined it to be all sufficient—She was deeply religious person and for her nursing was a vocation not a trade, but she was an educationist who believed that others besides Deaconesses and nuns could be good nurses—She also was a visionary and saw trained nursing as a secular career.

**"Our values give us the stars to navigate through life."**

# Chapter 17: Nurses Corner

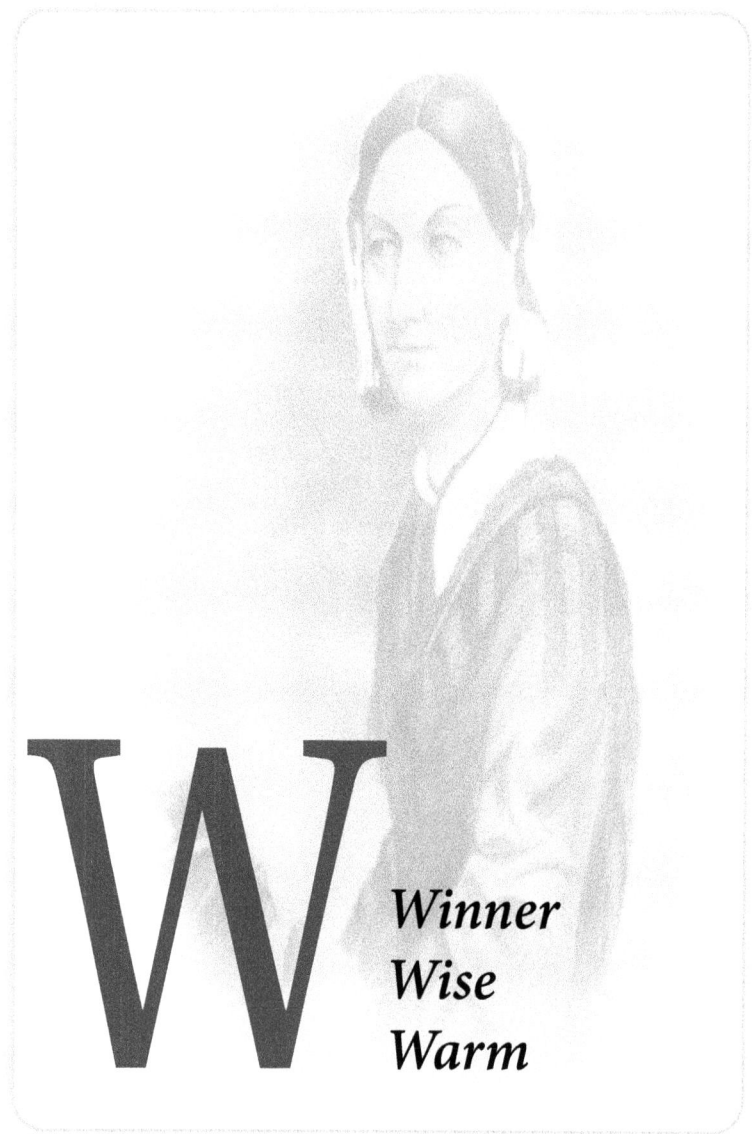

**W** *Winner*
*Wise*
*Warm*

> *"I work in the wards all day and write all night."*
> — *Florence Nightingale*

- "You ask me why I do no write something—I think one's feeling waste themselves in words, they ought all to be distilled into actions, which bring results."
- Bedside Nursing-Work for her was a passion a relaxant when she was weary of arguing with the purveyor, writing letters to ministers, listening to the complaints of a nurse, or coping with the ego of a doctor, she found strength at the bedside. Nightingale did not believe that God wanted or intended men to suffer, and she was fiercely convinced that the job of a nurse was to relieve the physical suffering of others, not to save her own soul by tending the sick.

**"Wise and humane management of the patient is the best safeguard against infection."**
— **Florence Nightingale**

**Chapter 17:** Nurses Corner

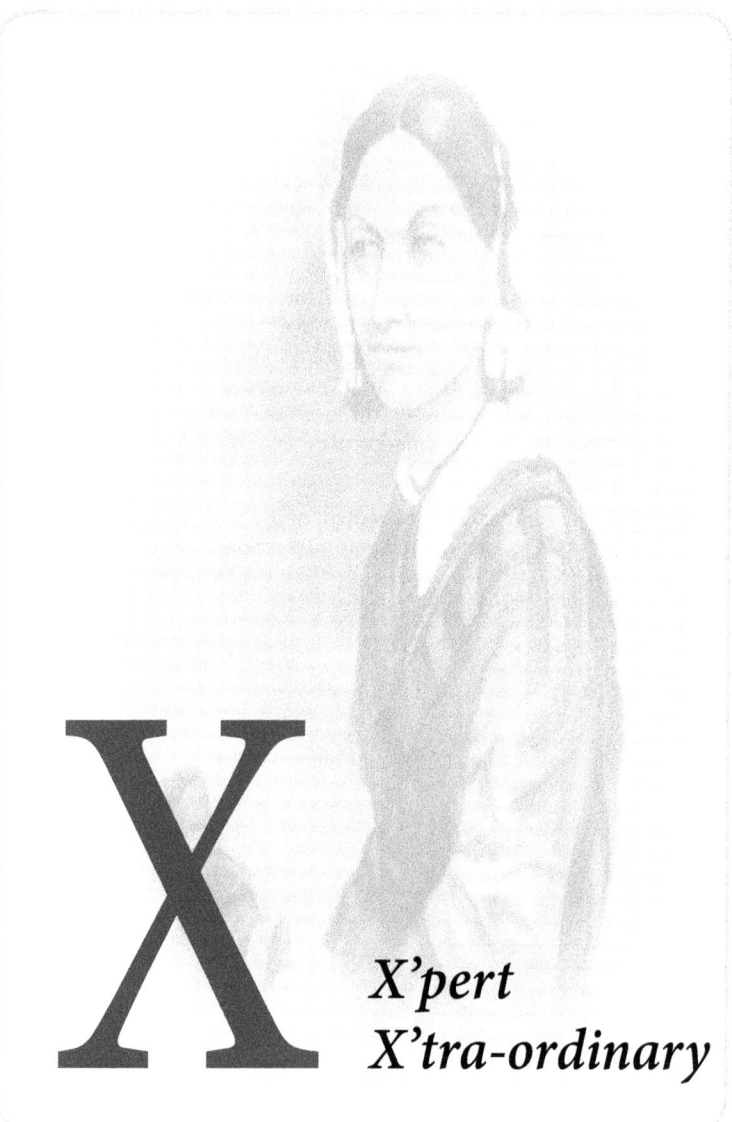

# X
## *X'pert*
## *X'tra-ordinary*

## Chapter 17: Nurses Corner

*X'cellence can be attained if you—"Care more than others think is wise; Risk more than others think is practical; Expect more than others think is possible."*

### We salute Florence Nightingale

- ❏ The Saint
- ❏ The Statistician
- ❏ The Writer
- ❏ The Linguist
- ❏ The Sanitarian and Hygienist
- ❏ The Nutritionist
- ❏ The Epidemiologist
- ❏ The Feminist
- ❏ The Hospital Reformer
- ❏ The Administrator
- ❏ The Educationist
- ❏ The Manager
- ❏ The Humanitarian and Hospital Reformer
- ❏ The Nurse

*"Legends never speak of themselves. They only do their work."*

**Chapter 17:** Nurses Corner

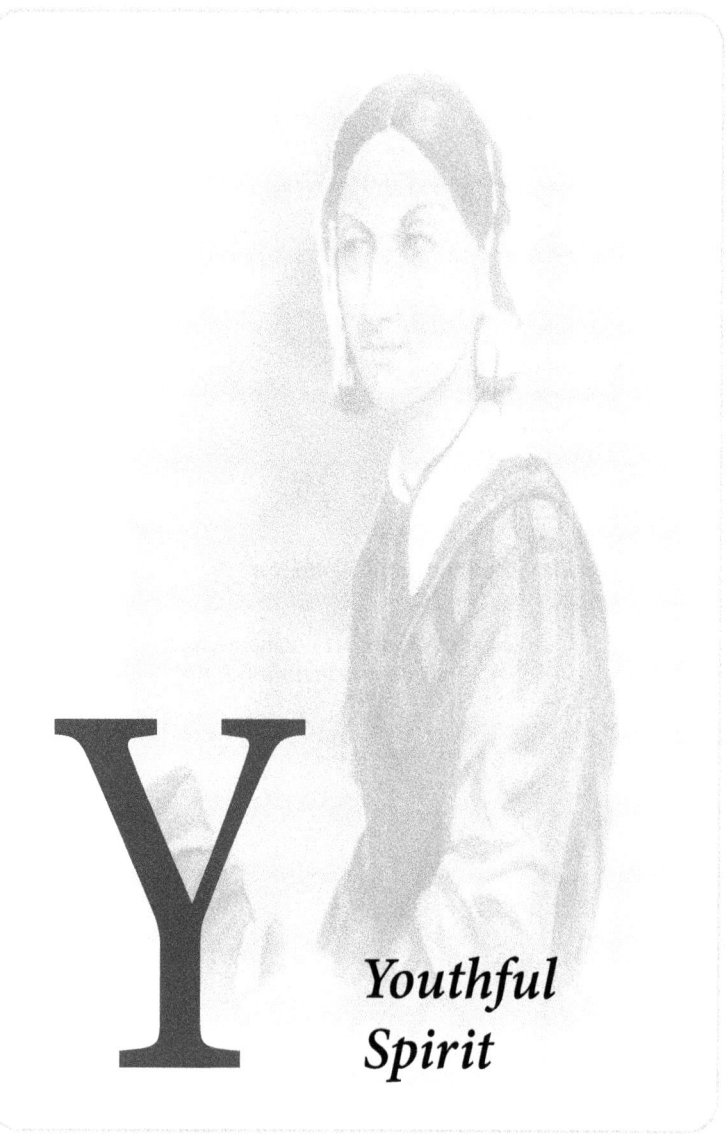

# Y
*Youthful Spirit*

## Chapter 17: Nurses Corner

*"It's not so much where you stand in life but in what direction you are moving."*

- She demonstrated untiring and endless effort for the betterment of patient care and hospital reforms.
- "Her entire youth was spent collecting the knowledge that would help her follow her "CALLING".
- In secret, she studied the reports of medical commissions, the pamphlets of sanitary authorities, the histories of hospitals and homes. She spent the intervals of the London season in workhouses.
- In February 1853, she traveled to France and visited all the city's public medical facilities.

**"Education is not the filling of a bucket but the lighting of fire".**

**She strongly believed that any education, any training must not only teach the mind but it must form the character.**

# Chapter 17: Nurses Corner

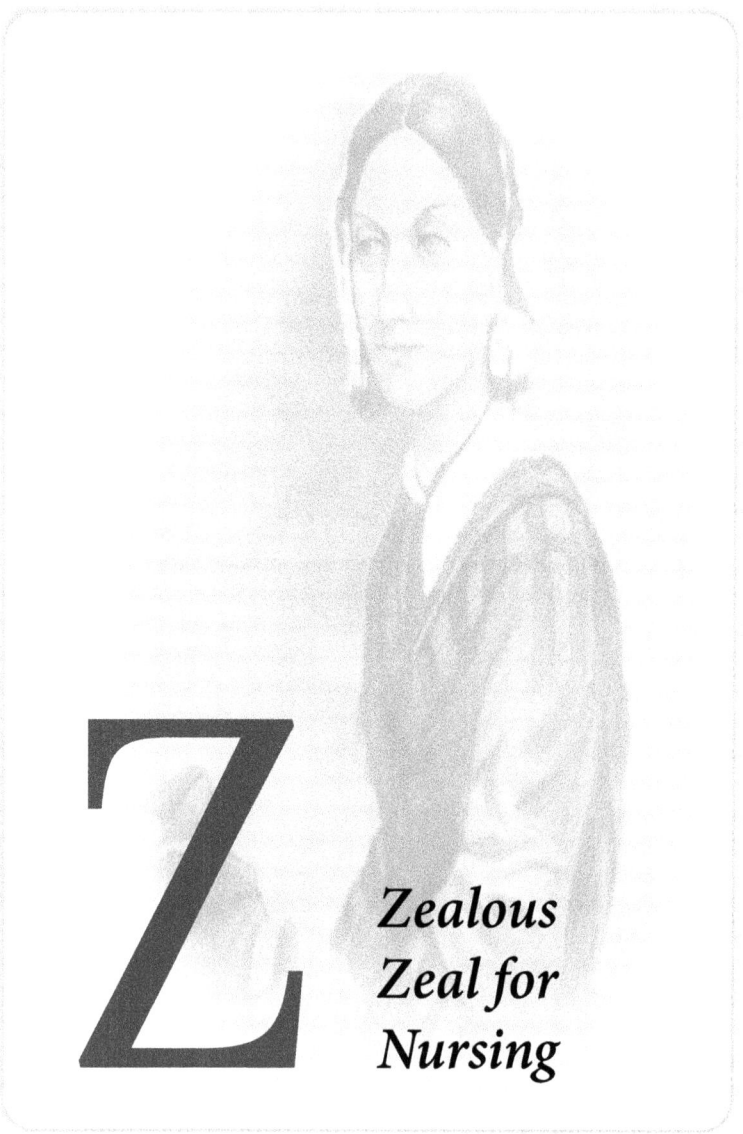

# Zealous Zeal for Nursing

*"Through zeal, knowledge is gotten, through lack of zeal, knowledge is lost."*

*Lord Buddha*

### Zealous
### Zeal for Nursing

- Florence Nightingale showed great energy and enthusiasm for nursing and hospital reforms she consistently strived to attain the best.
- "We can do no more for those who have suffered and died in their country's service; they need our help no longer; their spirits are with God who gave them. It remains to us to strive that their sufferings may not have been endured in vain—to endeavour so to learn from experience as to lessen such suffering in future by forethought and wise imagination."

"Enthusiasm is caught not taught."

"When shall we see a life full of enthusiasm, walking straight to its aim, flying home, as that bird is now, against the wind-with the calmness and the confidence of one who knows the laws of God and can apply them?"

*Florence Nightingale*

**Chapter 17:** Nurses Corner

## WHO ELSE BUT A NURSE

A stable 'head'
On responsible shoulders
Equipped with knowledge To counsel
And serve mankind!

Two strong, comforting 'Hands'
Full of dexterity and skill
Ever ready to serve,
To support, to nurture,
Nourish and heal the sick!

And A 'heart' of gold
Full of mercy, compassion and kindness
Ready to empathize,
Understand and console
Irrespective of creed or status!

Thus groomed she serves
In hospitals and in the community
An indispensable member of the human society
Who else, but a NURSE!

**P Biswas**

## SECTION B

## MAY 12TH INTERNATIONAL NURSES DAY

| Year | Theme |
|---|---|
| 1988 | Safe Motherhood |
| 1989 | School health |
| 1990 | Nurses and Environment |
| 1991 | Mental Health—Nurses in Action |
| 1992 | Healthy Aging |
| 1993 | Quality, Costs and Nursing |
| 1994 | Healthy Families for Healthy Nation |
| 1995 | Women's Health: Nurses Pave the Way |
| 1996 | Better Health through Nursing Research |
| 1997 | Healthy Young People = A Brighter Future |
| 1998 | Partnership for Community Health |
| 1999 | Celebrating Nursing's Past, Claiming the Future |
| 2000 | Nurses – Always There for You |
| 2001 | Nurses, Always There for You: United Against Violence |
| 2002 | Nurses Always There for You: Caring for Families |
| 2003 | Nurses: Fighting AIDS Stigma, Working for All |
| 2004 | Nurses: Working with the Poor; Against Poverty |
| 2005 | Nurses for Patients' Safety: Targeting Counterfeit Medicines and Substandard Medication |
| 2006 | Safe Staffing Saves Lives |
| 2007 | Positive Practice Environments: Quality Workplaces = Quality Patient Care |
| 2008 | Delivering Quality, Serving Communities: Nurses Leading Primary Health Care and Social Care |
| 2009 | Delivering Quality, Serving Communities: Nurses Leading Care Innovations |
| 2010 | Delivering Quality, Serving Communities: Nurses Leading Chronic Care |

| Year | Theme |
|---|---|
| 2011 | Closing the Gap: Increasing Access and Equity |
| 2012 | Closing the Gap: From Evidence to Action |
| 2013 | Closing the Gap: Millennium Development Goals |
| 2014 | Nurses: A Force for Change—A Vital Resource for Health |
| 2015 | Nurses: A Force for Change: Care Effective, Cost Effective |
| 2016 | Nurses: A Force for Change: Improving Health Systems' Resilience |
| 2017 | Nurses: A Voice to Lead—Achieving the Sustainable Development Goals |
| 2018 | Nurses: A Voice to Lead—Health is a Human Right |
| 2019 | Nurses: A Voice to Lead—Health for All |
| 2020 | Nurses: A Voice to Lead—Nursing the World to Health |
| 2021 | Nurses: A Voice to Lead—A Vision for Future Health care |
| 2022 | Nurses: Make a Difference |
| 2023 | Our Nurses. Our Future |

# CHAPTER 18

# Important Dates and Events

## 1820 BIRTH

In Florence city, the Nightingale has rented Villa Colombaia, a spacious and elegantly furnished villa located near the Porta Romana, just on the outskirts of the city. With its picturesque park and breathtaking views of the Duomo and Boboli Gardens, this villa holds a special significance—it was here that Florence Nightingale was born on May 12, 1820.

## JULY 1, 1820

Umiliana Pistelli (Balia) an Italian woman, signed a 3 year contract as nurse to Florence Nightingale.

Florence was encouraged by her mother to correspond with her nurse (when Florence was 8 years old).

## JULY 4, 1820

The baby was christened by Dr Trevor, Prebendary of Chester. Her given name was 'Florence'.

## 1830

Her father took over the education of his two daughters. From her father she learnt German, French, Latin, Italian, Greek, Mathematics, philosophy, politics and statistics (She received a 'man's education').

## 1837

'The calling'—She heard the voice of God calling her to do his work, she realized that her mission in life was to serve the sick.

## 1838

Florence visited Signora Pistelli met her "milk sister" Estella.

## 1844

Julia Howe recollects Florence asking her husband regarding nursing and her wish to become a nurse.

## 1844

7 years after her calling 'Florence Nightingale' asked Dr Howe (Julia Ward Howe's husband): "If I should determine to study nursing, and to devote my life to that profession, do you think it would be a dreadful thing?"

## 1845

She was anxious to go for training into Salisbury Hospital but the plan fizzled out.

## 1847

Florence Nightingale and her sister Parthenope attended the 1847 meeting of the British Association for the Advancement of Science at Oxford.

## 1851

Joins Kaiserswerth Institute in Germany.

## 1852

- Wrote a book titled 'Cassandra' but on advice of friends she never published this book.
- Studies Government Reports.
- Begins suggestions for thought, a religious treatise.

## AUGUST 1853–54

- Runs a hospital for sick Gentlewomen in London.
- Visits hospitals in Paris.

## 1854–56

Takes a group of nurses to Crimea.

## NOVEMBER 29, 1855

A public meeting was held in London which was destined to change the whole trend of nursing.

The meeting was presided over by the Commander-in-chief the Duke of Cambridge (Queen Victoria's first cousin) where the 'Nightingale Fund' was inaugurated, and within a short-time, after meetings had also been held in the provinces and Dominions, a sum of £ 44 ,000 was collected—The British soldier knew the value of women nurses in military hospitals and nearly £9,000 was subscribed by the Army.

The Nightingale training school, St. Thomas' London—thus came into being.

## FEBRUARY 1856

Peace was signed, but the work of the hospitals did not at once cease.

## JULY 27, 1856–57

Florence Nightingale, aunt Mai and Eliza Roberts traveled back to England on the steamer Danube-under assumed names.

## 1856 TO 1861

Royal Commission on the health of the Army—published (The commissions report was written in 1857) (for 5 years worked on the commission).

## OCTOBER 1856

She had a long interview with Queen Victoria and Prince Albert and the following year gave evidence to the 1857 Sanitary Commission. This eventually resulted in the formation of the Army Medical College.

## 1858

'Mortality of the British Army' a private edition. She produced 2000 copies of this book.

Notes on matters affecting the Health of the British Army. This was a confidential report to the Government, that Nightingale printed privately and sent to a number of people.

Became a member of the Royal Statistics Society.

## 1859

'England and Her soldiers' by Harriet Martineau—Florence encouraged Martineau to write the book about the war.

## 31ST MAY 1859

'Royal Commission on the Sanitary State of the Army in India' begins work.

## 1860

- Sidney Herbert created Lord Herbert.
- The Nightingale School for nurses set up at St. Thomas, London, (24th June 1860).
- 'Cassandra' privately printed.
- Writes paper on the importance of hospital statistics; read for her at International Statistical Congress.
- Notes on Nursing published.
- Suggestions for thought privately printed.

## 1861

Advices caring for the wounded in the America's civil war.

Deaths of Dr Alexander, Sidney Herbert, Arthur Hugh Clough, Prince Albert.

## 1862

- Publishes articles on Contagious Diseases Act.
- (1862 onwards) Engaged in work of India.

## 1863

Observations on the evidence contained in the stational reports submitted to her by the Royal Commission on the Sanitary State of the Army in India (Summary of Royal Commission Report). How people may live and not die in India. First read at the National Association for the Promotion of Social Science Congress, October 1863.

## 1864

- Writes to Thomas Longmore on the General convention 23rd July 1864.
- Henri Dunant's speech on Florence Nightingale at the Geneva convention (August 1864).
- The cause of reform in work house nursing (engaged her time and energies).

## 1864–68

Work with war office on India Sanitary Reform; with William Rathbone on workhouse nursing.

## 1867

Suggestions on the subject of providing, training and organizing nurses for the sick poor in workhouse infirmaries.

## 1870

Took up the question of district nursing.
She was elected member of the Bengal Social Sciences Association.

## 1871

St. Thomas Hospital was reopened (in its present position).

## 1873

Two essays on the laws of the moral world were published by Froude in Frasers Magazine for May and July titles were:
1. "A note of interrogation" and
2. "A sub note of interrogation: what will our religion be in 1999?

## 1874

Honorary member of the American Statistical Association.

## 1883

Received Royal Red Cross award from Queen Victoria.

## 1893

She dedicated a lecture on 'Sick Nursing and Health Nursing' to Princes Christian which was read at the Chicago Exhibition of women's work.

## 1895

In later life suffered from poor health went blind.

## 1897

The year of Queen Victoria's Diamond Jubilee—"The Victorian Era Exhibition was held which included a section representing the progress of trained nursing and (that) it was planned round Miss Nightingale.

## 1907

Awarded 'Order of Merit' by the British Crown.

## 1908

Freedom of the city of London was conferred on her.

## 13TH AUG. 1910

Died in her sleep.

## HER VIEWS ON DEATH

- "I am sure it is an immense activity."

  Florence Nightingale

  (She considered death not rest but activity)
- "A human being does not cease to exist at death. It is change, not destruction, which takes place."

  Florence Nightingale

**Death be not proud**
She left instructions that after her death her body was to be given for dissection. There was to be no state funeral, no burial in West-Minister Abbey partly her wishes were fulfilled, she was buried in the little churchyard of East Wellow next to her parents. The monument on her grave reads:

"FN Born May 1820
Died 13th August, 1910".

"One short sleep past,
We wake eternally,
Death shall be no more,
Death thou shalt die."

**John Donne, 1572–1631**

# CHAPTER 19

# Priceless Pearls: Quotations of Miss Florence Nightingale

Let us each and all realize the importance of our influence on others—stand shoulder to shoulder and not alone in a good cause.

It may seem a strange principle to enunciate as the very first requirement in a hospital that it should do the sick no harm (1859).

Let us be anxious to do well, not for selfish praise, but to honour and advance the cause, the work we have taken up (as nurses).

The very essence of all good organization is that everybody should do her or his work in such a way as to help and not hinder everyone else's work.

Nursing is an art; and if it is to be made an art, requires as exclusive a devotion, as hard a preparation as any painter's or sculptor's work; for what is the having to do with dead canvas or cold marble, compared with having to do with the living body—the temple of Gods spirit—it is one of the fine arts. I have almost said, the finest of fine arts.

For us who nurse, our nursing is a thing, which, unless in it we are making progress every year, every month, every week, take my word for it, we are going back.

Let each founder train as many in her/his spirit as he/she can. Their pupils will in their turn be founder also.

## Chapter 19: Priceless Pearls: Quotations of Miss Florence Nightingale

"Let whoever is Incharge keep this simple question in her head (not how can I always do this right thing myself) but how can I provide for this right thing to always be done."

'Asceticism is the trifling of an enthusiast with his power, a puerile coquetting with his selfishness or his vanity, in the absence of any sufficiently great object to employ the first or overcome the last' (1857).

'I can stand out the war with any man.'

The honour does not lie in putting on Nursing like your uniform. Honour lies in loving perfection, consistency, and in working hard for it: in being ready to work patiently: ready to say not "How clever I am" but "I am not yet worthy; and I will live to deserve to be called a Trained Nurse."

No man, not even a doctor, ever gives any other definition of what a nurse should be than this devoted and obedient. Would do just as well for a porter. It might even do for a horse. It would not do for a policeman (1859).

For what is Mysticism? Is it not the attempt to draw near to God, not by rites or ceremonies, but by inward disposition? Is it not merely a hard word for the Kingdom of Heaven is within? Heaven is neither a place nor a time (1873).

"Ingenuity and perseverance (and these really constitute the good nurse) might save more lives than we wot of."

"But if you cannot get the habit of observation one way or another you had better give up being a nurse, for it is not your calling, however, kind and anxious you may be."

'I stand at the altar of the murdered men, and while I live, I fight their cause'. (1865)

## Chapter 19: Priceless Pearls: Quotations of Miss Florence Nightingale

"The progressive world is necessarily divided into two classes—those who take the best of what there is and enjoy it—those who wish for something better and try to create it."

"Were there none who were discontented with what they have, the world would never reach anything better."

"The dreams of youth have become a proverb."

"When shall we see a life full of steady enthusiasm, walking straight to its aim, flying home, as that bird is now, against the wind—with the calmness and the confidence of one who knows the laws of God and can apply them?"

"Religion is not devotion but work and suffering for the love of God."

"There will be no heaven, unless we makes it."

"The mystical state is the essence of common sense."

"Must we not 'Possess' God here, if we want to 'Possess' Him hereafter."

"Desire for personal salvation is not religion."

"Never has God let me feel weariness of active life, but only anxiety to get on. Now in old age I never wish to be relieved from new work, but only to have it do it."

## Chapter 19: Priceless Pearls: Quotations of Miss Florence Nightingale

"The way to live with God is to live ideas—not merely to think about ideas but to do and suffer for them."

"Women are unable to see that it requires wisdom as well as self-denial to establish a new work." (1866)

"I have thought I could work better, even for other women, off the stage than on it."

"Everything has gone from my life except pain." (1874)

"I have no time. It is 14 years to this very day that I entered upon work which has never left me ten minutes leisure, not even to be ill. And I am obliged not to give my name where I cannot give my work."

"Oh that I could do something for India."
(Private Note 1878)

"O happiness—like the Bread Fruit Tree, what a corrupter of human nature thou art!"

"Nursing has to nurse living bodies and spirit. It cannot be tested by public examination, though it may be tested by current supervision."

"Those who undertake the work of aiding the sick and wounded must not be sentimental enthusiasts but downright lovers of hard work."

"I attribute my success to this: I never gave or took an excuse."

"A human being does not cease to exist at death. It is change, not destruction, which takes place."

"How very little can be done under the spirit of fear."

"I am sure it is an immense activity (she considered death not rest, but activity)."

"There are things worse than death."

"An eternity of silence seems too short to rest me." 1876

"It must be a home—a place of character, habits and intelligence, as well as of acquiring knowledge." (Regarding a Nursing School 1875)

"Oh God, let me not sink in these perplexities but give me a great cause to do and die for (Private Note)."

"All our actions, all our words, all our thoughts, the food on which they are to live and have their being, is the indwelling presence of God, the union with God."

"I have never been used to influence people except by leading in work; and to have to influence them by talking and writing is hard. A more dreadful thing than being cut short by death is being cut short by life in a paralyzed state." (Letter to Clarkey 1875)

"I do so believe every tear one sheds waters some good thing into life." (1844)

**Chapter 19:** Priceless Pearls: Quotations of Miss Florence Nightingale

"All restless anxiety is from want of trust in God". (Feb. 1846)

"Apprehension, uncertainty, waiting, expectation, fear of surprise, do a patient more harm than any exertion." (1844)

"Unnecessary noise, then, is the most cruel absence of care which can be inflicted either on the sick or well." (1844)

"How different would be the heart for the work, and how different would be the success, if we learnt our work as a serious study, and followed it out steadily as a professional."

# CHAPTER 20

## Strange but True

Florence Nightingale's period of greatest activity and achievement (1857–72) was exactly the period when she was bedridden, in an agony of pain, exhausted, depressed and apparently on the edge of death.

### "The Great Serenifer"
For Nightingale, nursing was a practical imperative and a spiritual exercise, providing a nexus of body and soul that gave her the deepest satisfaction. It was, in her own words, "The great serenifer."

### Work for her was a passion, a relaxant.
When she was weary of arguing with the purveyor, writing letters to ministers, listening to the complaints of a nurse, or coping with the ego of a doctor, she found strength at the bed-side. Nightingale did not believe that God wanted or intended men to suffer, and she was fiercely convinced that the job of a nurse was to relieve the physical suffering of others, not to save her own soul by tending the sick.

She wrote to a rebellious nurse on April 22nd, 1869 "Do you think I should have succeeded in doing anything if I had kicked and resisted and resented?................. I have been shut out of hospitals into which I had been ordered by the Commander-in-Chief, obliged to stand outside the door in the snow until night, have been refused rations for as much as 10 days at a time for the nurses I had brought by superior command."

# CHAPTER 21

# Apprehensions

She was only human, her apprehensions, mental exhaustion, despair and pain were many; despair alternated with self-reproach, failures pursued and haunted her; mistakes and disasters added to her pain.

"Everything has gone from my life except pain."
**(Letter to Clarkey 1874)**

- "Oh God, let me not sink in these perplexities but give me a great cause to do and die for."
(Recorded in a private note)
- One night, when she got up from sleep, the shadow cast by the night light on the wall reminded her of Scutari........ "Am I she who once stood on that Crimea height?"
- "There is no longer any consecutive path growing out of my own acts, only a succession of disjointed lives and disconnected events."
- "Latterly I have been so broken up and broken down. Nothing solaces me so much as to write upon the Laws of the Moral World."
- In February 1874 Quetelet, originator of the science of statistics, died—she pondered—how much he had achieved compared to her....... what makes the difference between man and women? Quetelet did his work and I am so disturbed by my family that I can't do mine."
- "My life now is an unlike my hospital life when I was concerned with the souls and bodies of men as reading a cookery book is unlike a good dinner."
(Letter to Rev. Mother Bermondsey 1864)
- "Oh to be turned back to this petty stagnant stifling life at Embley, which has done to death so many of the best with whom I began life."
(Private note 1872)

## Chapter 21: Apprehensions

- "I am stifled by dirty anxious cares and sordid defensive business; like the maid of all work who has to wipe her dirty hands on her dirtier apron before she can touch clean people" 1872.
- "Oh my Creator, thou knowest that through all these twenty horrible years I have been supported by the belief that I was working with Thee who were bringing every one, even our poor nurses to perfection."
- 1852—"My present life is suicide My God what will become of me?"

> "Yet I would spare no pang, would wish no torture less the more that anguish racks, the earlier it will bless."

- "Give us back our suffering, we cry to heaven in our hearts—suffering rather than indifferentism; for out of nothing comes nothing. But out of suffering may come the cure. *Better have pain than paralysis!* A hundred struggle and drown in the breakers. One discovers the new world. But rather, ten times rather, die in the surf, heralding the way to that new world, than stand idly on the shore!"

# CHAPTER 22

# India—Florence Nightingale's Vision and Contributions

"She refused to view India as a conquest: the enormous responsibility of India had been placed by providence in the hands of the British people as a scared trust, and the object of the British official should be to work for the time when the country could be handed back to the people of India endowed with the greatest blessings of Western Civilization—health."

Strange but true—She had never been to India, her knowledge was a paper knowledge, yet 3/4th of the sanitation and improvements in India were due to her.

All papers dealing with Indian sanitary questions were sent to her for her comments.
- The annual report of the sanitary department.
- The Indian sanitary annual was produced under her direction.
- She drafted the "Introductory memorandum" to the sanitary annual commenting on the years progress.

**She corresponded with:**
- President of the Madras Sanitary Commission
- The doctors who sent reports on the sanitary condition of jails
- With Secretaries of each Presidential Sanitary Commission.

"The first possibility of rural cleanliness lies in water supply."
**Florence Nightingale**

Miss Nightingale was convinced that the best way to develop sanitary education, in England as in India, was to use the village as a unit. And she insisted, "The work must be personal", the Health Missioners were not to lecture the village women but to work with them.

In 1872, the engineers to the Municipality of Calcutta came to see her—the city of Calcutta which was growing and was overcrowded was in urgent need of a drainage scheme and a pure water supply. After examining the plans she wrote a detailed memorandum to Sir, George Campbell, Lieutenant Governor of Bengal. The difficulties were overcome.

> She never visited India, but so great was her knowledge of Indian sanitary army affairs that no important government official left for India without seeing her.

> She directed the purification of the Madras water system from her bedroom in South Street London.

- In 1870, she was elected an honorary member of the Bengal Social Science Association, which was largely composed of native gentleman. In collaboration with Sir Bartle Frere, she wrote a paper addressed to the village elder on Indian sanitation which was read at their proceedings. The Association had it translated into Bengali and other Indian dialects and it was widely circulated.

> "She was the only human being who had ever mastered the Bengal land purchase system."
>
> **Sir John Lawrence**

- In 1868 (approx year), Florence Nightingale realized that nothing could be done in India until India was fed.

> "Famine is the constant condition of the people."
>
> **Florence Nightingale**

Hence irrigation works became Miss Nightingale first aim for India.
- She did a lot of work for the improvement of the barracks and sanitary measures for the English army stationed in India.
- In 1870, war was declared between Germany and France and Miss Nightingale was asked to take control, but she was not prepared to stop her present work—she considered her Indian work more important as one author puts it.

"One laborious memorandum on sanitation in India affected the lives of millions on whom, even if her health allowed, she could never turn her back to become the Lady with the Lamp once more."

**Cecil Woodham Smith**

But the world would not leave her alone and she accomplished a lot of work for the 'British Red Cross Aid Society' during the German-France war.

Observations on the Evidence contained in the stational reports submitted to her by the Royal Commission on the Sanitary State of the Army in India (Summary of Royal Commission Report). How people may live and not die in India. First read at the National Association for the Promotion of Social Science Congress, October 1863.

Works with War Office on Indian Sanitary Reform; with William Rathbone on Workhouse nursing (1864–68).

# CHAPTER 23

# Caring is Active Prayer

## SPECIAL FEATURE

101 ways to understand what *'caring'* and caring behavior means in Nursing (1820–1910).

> Caring is touching grace itself

> Caring is everything nothing matters but caring (Baron F von Hugel)

- **Caring** is being willing and able to nurture others (Leininger).
- **Caring** is one of life's essential ingredients: It may be the most essential ingredient (EO Bevis).
- **Caring** is the basis of nursing.
- **Caring** is not an abstract concept but is demonstrated by nurses in various ways.
- **Caring** is commitment.
- **Caring** is interpreted by many as being a moral imperative. Through caring for other human beings, ultimately human dignity is protected, enhanced, and preserved.
- **Caring** is the very heart of nursing.
- **Caring** is very personal, and thus its expression will differ for each client.
- **Caring** means responding to others as unique individuals, sensing their emotions, and accepting them as they are unconditionally.
- **Caring** preserves human dignity in a cure - dominated healthcare system.
- One of the foundational concepts of caring as a science is: **Caring for the whole person** also known as **'transpersonal caring'**, holistic nursing. We also refer to it as 'high-touch nursing'.
- **Caring** is creating an environment of hope and trust, understanding the meaning of the experience to the patient and family.

- **Caring** means 'being with' the patient not just 'doing things' for the patient.
- **Caring** is the moral ideal that guides nurses through the care giving process, and knowledgeable caring is the highest form of commitment (Watson 1995).
- **Caring** involves being assertive and responsible.
- **Caring** is situation-specific.
- **Caring** includes an ongoing commitment to sharpening knowledge and skills to identify care needs and nursing actions that will bring about positive change while protecting and enhancing human dignity.
- **Caring** emphasizes a patient's individuality.

Caring is important not only to the practice of nursing but also for the existence of humankind.

- **Caring** is central to the nursing practice.
- **Caring** actualizes a cherished value in nursing: the individualization of client care.
- **Caring** is at the heart of a nurses ability to work with people in a respectful and therapeutic way.
- True **caring** emphasizes the nurses enabling presence.
- The most completely human thing about nurses is **'caring'**
- **Caring** is 'touching grace itself.
- **Caring** is the 'why' of nursing.
- **Caring** means sharing the patient's experiences, sharing faith and sharing life—life which struggles for recovery, for normalcy.
- **Caring** makes a connection with another human being and breaks down the alienation that not caring creates.
- All persons are **caring,** although not all actions are caring.
- **Caring** means caring for the patient, the patient's family, patient's relatives and all significant others.
- **Caring** is delivering quality holistic care to all persons without discrimination.

## CARING INCLUDES EVERYONE

- **Caring** means, setting aside all negative feelings, not criticizing but rendering holistic care to all.

- **Caring** means talking to the patient's family, relatives, teaching them, also caring enough for their concerns, fears and stress.
- **Caring** is providing the most valuable kind of care to the needy and sick.
- **Caring** is a personal as well as a professional behavior.
- **Caring** means, helping your co-workers and colleagues to perform and to give in their best.
- Meeting the challenges of caring for another human being is the highest form of **caring**.
- **Caring** is meeting the needs of the sick and suffering fellow being.
- **Caring** is bringing into every interaction, compassion and responsible behavior and high ideals of caring and nursing.
- **Caring** is using healing arts with skill, knowledge, compassion and understanding, promptly and as and when required.
- **Caring** is respecting the patient as a person.
- **Caring** means being a sensitive and compassionate listener.
- **Caring** is creating healing environments' for persons under your care.
- **Caring** means helping the patient to empower himself/herself by giving them the right information, teaching them needed skills that make it possible for them to take control of their own lives and health.
- **Caring** therefore means creating empowering conditions for the people under your care.
- **Caring** is trusting your patient and helping the patient to achieve desired health goals.
- **Caring** calls for a philosophy of moral commitment toward protecting human dignity and preserving humanity (Watsm 1988).
- **Caring** means being both a high-tech and a high-touch nurse and giving care with responsibility, with empathy and in an ethical way as and when required.
- **Caring** is nursing the sick.
- **Caring** improves human conditions and life processes.
- **Caring** means meeting the patient's perceived health care needs.
- **Caring** is person-focused and nursing-focused care.
- **Caring** is a common bond of persons situated in a state of being.
- **Caring** is helping individuals to reach normalcy and independence that is essential to nursing. (Patricia Benner and Judith Wrubel 1989)

## Chapter 23: Caring is Active Prayer

- **Caring** is the ability to develop trusting professional relationships with both patients and colleagues, relationships which enhance the worth and dignity of all concerned.
- **Caring** is respecting every single persons individuality.
- **Caring** is understanding and being aware of the expression of life around you.

Caring is to respect your own body and the body of all under your care as the 'Temple of God'.

- **Caring** means to respect and support the religious or spiritual needs of the person under your care.
- **Caring** is consistent manner from shift to shift, day to day—with the help of responsible communication amongst care givers.
- **Caring** is a motivating force for people to become nurses.
- **Caring** is being able to make a +ve, healing difference in the lives of people.
- **Caring** is creating an environment in the workplace which is conducive to healing.
- **Caring** is always specific and relational for each nurse-client encounter.
- **Caring** involves mutual give and take that develops as nurse and client begin to know and care for one another.
- **Caring** is knowing your patient and undertaking the patient's perception of illness.
- **Caring** is the skillful and gentle performance of nursing procedures and it promotes security.
- **Caring** is providing a sense of closeness—its being there and being with the patient.
- **Caring** is the fundamental essence of nursing care, underpinning nursing knowledge and practice (Madeleine Leininger, 1978). It is the innate drive to extend compassion and support to individuals who are unwell, vulnerable, or experiencing distress.
- **Caring** is understanding and accepting the essential dignity of every individual.
- **Caring** is honoring the life of the spirit (atman).
- **Caring** is providing basic care and creating order and a sense of community, even in the most extreme and violent settings.
- **Caring** is to alleviate suffering and pain, to give health and hope also to give self-respect.

- **Caring** is believing that everyone deserves a fair chance at a healthy life; it means helping all persons to enjoy their basic Human Rights.
- **Caring** is to seek out the most vulnerable people and to serve them.
- **Caring** is to approach the patient from a holistic perspective, it stresses on the importance of provider-patient partnerships and respectful communication.
- **Caring** is to address the biopsychosocial and spiritual needs of patients who are receiving nursing care.
- **Caring** is voicing through action not words alone.
- **Caring** is promotion of health and hope.
- **Caring** is fighting discrimination it's giving health and care with compassion and responsibility.
- **Caring** means reaching out to those most in need.
- **Caring** is to advocate, to also innovate and above all to care.
- **Caring** is 'being there' when life begins and when it ends

>'When Life is Born I Welcome it,
>My Hands, The First to Hold it;
>> I Serve
>>
>> I Nurture
>>
>> I Nourish
>>
>> I Care
>>
>> I AM A NURSE

- **Caring** is bringing alive the essence of humanity that forms us all.
- **Caring** is being a 'healing presence' in people's lives.
- **Caring** is harboring a responsibility to other human beings.
- **Caring** is the power to make a difference in another persons life (the one cared for).
- **Caring** is a bond that ties (humanity) people and nurses together.
- **Caring** is one of the most fundamental expressions of human concern.
- **Caring** is to provide social support to a patient who is alone without kith or kin.
- **Caring** is building a relationship of trust and respect with people, even if they are culturally or economically different.
- **Caring** is nursing and vice versa.

## Chapter 23: Caring is Active Prayer

Caring is managing technology and at the same time providing, the 'human face of health care'.

- **Caring** is protecting life, saving life and also making life easier.
- **Caring** is humankind's commitment to care for all those in need for care. It also means caring for one another.
- **Caring** is providing a honest human touch to lives in times of great distress.
- **Caring** is creating the conditions that will give people everywhere a fair chance at living healthy life.

Caring means—caring for the individuals body—even after the patients' death, with respect, gentleness and love.

**'CARING IS VOCING THROUGH ACTION NOT WORDS ALONE'.**

*"Nursing is not an adventure ............... as some have now supposed — It is very serious, delightful thing, like life, requiring training experience, devotion, a power of accumulating, instead of losing ............... all these things".*

Florence Nightingale 1897

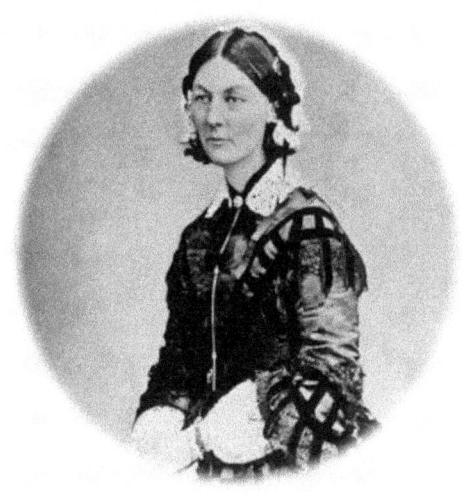

1820–1910

## Chapter 23: Caring is Active Prayer

**Caring and nursing are two sides of the same coin and complement each other and are the hallmarks of the caring profession.**

Your agenda as a Nurse **today** and **everyday** is—

### 'Caring Care'
### *The Caring Rainbow*

The seven colors of Nursing

**VIOLET:** Richness of the soul, immortality

**INDIGO:** Comforting presence enabling presence

**BLUE:** Knowledge and understanding infinite kindness

**GREEN:** Everlasting life

**YELLOW:** Aura, faith, enlightment, light, joy, friendliness reaching out creativity

**ORANGE:** Spirituality, intuition, focused, goal-oriented action and WISDOM

**RED:** LOVE OF GOD: Power, force, vitality, passion to serve, life's vital force

**REMEMBER ALWAYS**
At the heart of nursing is the human being.

## POEM

GIVE ME WINGS
of
Knowledgeable
Caring
And.... I'll Learn
to fly;
Beston on me
YOUR divine Grace
and... strength
as 'wind'
AND
STAY BY MY
SIDE....,
AND
I'LL SOAR HIGH

**Pushpa Biswas**

# CHAPTER 24

## Conclusion

The setting sun said:

> "Who will take up my work?
> The world heard this and
> Yet remained responseless
>     like a picture
> There was an earthen lamp,

It said:
> "Lord! I will exert myself to my utmost"

—Rabindranath Tagore

Like the earthen lamp we as nurses have work to do lets move forward—let's grow together, let's endeavor to lift 'Nursing' to the heights Florence Nightingale desired, that would be the greatest homage to the 'Lady with the Lamp.' Let's pledge to commit ourselves to quality.

## Chapter 24: Conclusion

Dear Reader,

Now that you are at this end of the book, your curiosity to know more about this enigmatic personality must have been aroused and it is for this reason that an effort has been made to arrange information in an easy reading format for you. This book has been also compiled to encourage student nurses, in fact all nurses to learn and know about the founder of Modern Nursing Miss Florence Nightingale.

All readers must have felt that a lot more can be added to each chapter, do start 'now' this book has been compiled painstakingly and should have a place reserved in every nurses book shelf.

All suggestions are welcome.
With best wishes and prayers.

**P Biswas**

# Further Reading

1. Dunbar VM, Dolan MB. Notes on nursing: what it is, and what it is not. New York: Dover publications, 1969.
2. Seymer Lucy Ridgely. A general history of nursing. London: Faber and Faber, 1949.
3. www.en.wikipedia.org/wiki/Florence Nightingale. Accessed on 15th Mar, 2009.
4. www.spartacus,schoolnet.co.uk/REnightingale.htm Accessed on 17th Mar, 2009.
5. www.worldofbiography.com/9062-Florence%20 Nightingale/quotations.htm Accessed on 26th Mar, 2009.

# Index

## A

Aboriginal races, protection of  11
Active prayer, caring  128
Administrations  11
Agatha and Christie, biographies of  15
Appointed course  47
Army Medical Board  23
Athena  43

## B

Barrack hospital  45
Bed
    and bedding  13
    spacing between  49
British museum  11

## C

Calling  3
Caring includes everyone  129
Cassandra trojan prophetess  27
Central kitchen  24
Chattering hopes and advices  13
Cholera  19, 23
Clean laundry  49
Coxcomb  6, 43
Crimea's dread shores  39
Crimean
    fever  23
    mission  35
    war  36
Critical thinking  44, 50
    skills  34

## D

Dates and events, important  109
Dysentery  23

## E

End of war  35

## F

Family  30
Father daughter special bond  1
Financial independence, importance of  17
Florence
    brilliancy  3
    childhood  1
    sister  46
Florence nightingale  10
    caring educationist  17
    day  17
    educationist  16
    epidemiologist  23
    feminist  26
    honor of  44
    humanitarian, nurse  32
    intellectual self-confidence  15
    interest, part of  7
    John Sutherland wrote to  46
    life  6
    linguist  15
    notes on nursing  12
    nurse
        administrator  22
        manager  22
    nutritionist  24
    saint  4
    sanitarian, hygienist and hospital
        reformer  19
    statistician  6
    time  7
    tribute to  40
    vision and contributions  125
    work  41
    writer  8
    writings  9

Food 13
    taking 13
Fresh air 49

## G

Gardens, acres of 1
Gender-related difficulties 26
Glorious tributes 36
God's creatures 4
God's law of healing 34
Great skill and efficiency 34

## H

Health 11
    care 32
    chance of 32
    of houses 12
Heart 69
Home sister 18
Hospitals 11
Human immune system 49
Hygienic measures 49

## I

International Nurses Day 107

## K

Kaiserswerth her spiritual home 10

## L

Lady with lamp 38
Letters 45
Light 13

## M

Malaria 19
Mathematics 2
Matron's direction 18
Military
    character 47
    system 47
Minding baby 10

Miss Florence nightingale,
    quotations of 116
Moral activity 29

## N

Needlework 6
Nightingale's
    letters 41
    plan 16
    pledge 37
    school 11, 17, 18
    system 18
Noise 12
Nurse
    corner 51
    shortages 34
    who else but a 106
Nursing 11
    alphabets of 51
    knowledge, focus of 12
    notes on 8, 9
    practice, boundaries of 12
    sick, methods of 18
    student of 12
Nutritious food 24

## P

Particular vocation 47
Patient's
    nutrition 25
    personal clothing, regular
        change of 49
    rights, respect for 44, 50
Personal cleanliness 13
Petty management 12
Philosophy 2
Pie 6
    chart 6
Politics 2
Pre and postwar period 34
Preventive medicine 10
Privacy, providing of 50
Public health, history of 20

## R

Red cross  36
    movement  42
Registration statistics  7
Regular digestible  24
Remittance scheme  22, 50
Rhine' first work  9
Rooms and walls, cleanliness of  13
Royal commission  10
Russian prisoner  39

## S

Sanitations  11
Scar tissue, formation of  49
Science  2
Separate sponge cloth, use of  49
Sick
    observation of  14
    population  32
    soldiers, wounded  33
    ward, workhouse  33
Sidney Herbert's tribute  41
Skin, cleanliness of  49
Spiritual home  28
Steady enthusiasm  28
Strange but true  122

## T

Tell miss nightingale  42
Theoretical teaching  18
Therapeutic diet  49
Therapeutic environment  49
Thoughtful stillness, moments of  3
Trained nurse  69, 117

## V

Variety  13
Varna fever  23
Ventilation  12
    good  49

## W

Warming  12
Western Sanitary Commission  36
Woman
    dream  28
    education  2
    **passion**  29
    **suffrage**  11